Voices from the Heart

Inspirations for a Compassionate Future

edited by Eddie and Debbie Shapiro

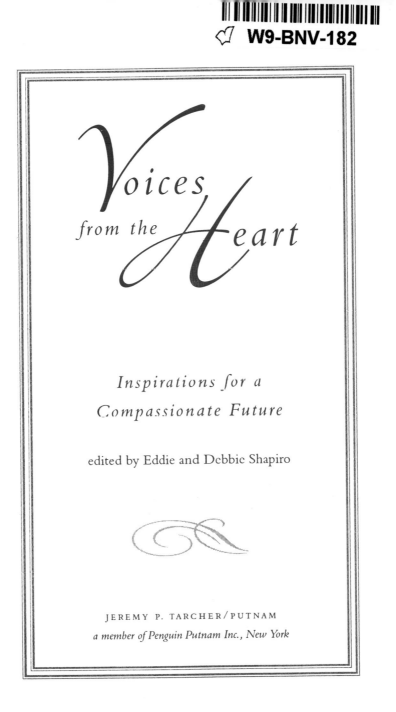

JEREMY P. TARCHER/PUTNAM
a member of Penguin Putnam Inc., New York

Most Tarcher/Putnam books are available at special quantity discounts for bulk purchases for sales promotions, premiums, fund-raising, and educational needs. Special books or book excerpts also can be created to fit specific needs. For details, write Putnam Special Markets, 375 Hudson Street, New York, NY 10014.

Photograph of the Dalai Lama © Taikan Usui. Photograph of Yoko Ono © 1992 Jayne Wexler, Courtesy of Lenono Photo Archive. Photograph of Satish Kumar © Kate Mount, Devon, England. Photograph of Cathrine Sneed © 1992 J. Patrick Forden. All Rights Reserved. Photograph of Stephen Levine © William Abranowitz. Photograph of Anita Roddick © Gregg Gorman. Photograph of Mikhail Gorbachev © Associated Press AP/Wide World Photos. Photograph of Thich Nhat Hanh by Karen Hagen Liste. Photograph of Anne Bancroft © Jeff Bowden, LMPA.

Jeremy P. Tarcher/Putnam
a member of
Penguin Putnam Inc.
375 Hudson Street
New York, NY 10014
www.penguinputnam.com

The Library of Congress had cataloged the hardback edition as follows:
Voices from the heart : a compassionate call for responsibility / edited
by Eddie and Debbie Shapiro.

p.   cm.
ISBN 0-87477-935-9 (alk. paper)
1. Spiritual life.   I. Shapiro, Eddie, date.   II. Shapiro,
Debbie, date.

BL624.V64   1998   98-4005 CIP
ISBN 0-87477-984-7 (trade paperback edition)

Printed in the United States of America
1   2   3   4   5   6   7   8   9   10

This book is printed on acid-free paper. ∞

BOOK DESIGN BY RALPH FOWLER

Voices from the Heart

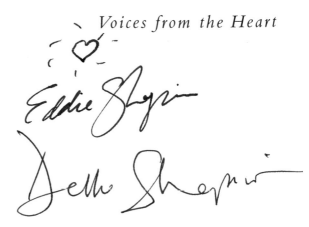

Eddie Shapiro

Debbie Shapiro

Acknowledgments

Our thanks go first to our publisher, Joel Fotinos, who caught the vision with such enthusiasm and friendship, and our editor, David Groff, for his careful attention to detail. Also thanks to Kristen Giorgio, our publicist. Our appreciation goes to Fred Matser for his interview with Mikhail Gorbachev, and to Stephen Batchelor for his interview with Sulak Sivaraksa. Our gratitude goes to Mel Bricker at Matthew Fox's office, Gwilym Jones and Helen O'Connell at Glenys Kinnock's office, and Bea at Rama Vernon's office. Rachel Naomi Remen's contribution is adapted from "Spirit: Resource for Healing," printed in *Noetic Science Review,* Autumn 1988; the stories are adapted by permission of the publisher from *Kitchen Table Wisdom: Stories That Heal,* by Rachel Naomi Remen, M.D. (New York: Riverhead Books, 1996). Thich Nhat Hanh's contribution is edited from *Love in Action: Writings on Nonviolent Social Change* (Berkeley: Parallax Press, 1993).

Our deep thanks and gratitude go to Susan Mears for her vision, editorial comments, and advice; John Clamp for transcribing so many diverse voices; and Christopher Titmuss for giving this project so much of his time and energy. To Joanne Sawicki, Katie Thompson, Jill Dawson, Satish Kumar, Anne and Richard Bancroft, Nirmala Heriza, Mark, Nané, Jenny, Liz, Joani, Theo, Julie, Jim, Demaris, and Mary, we thank you all for your love and support.

*Dedicated to the
benefit of all beings*

Contents

PART THREE
HEALING AND WHOLENESS   149

PART FOUR
ECONOMY AND ECOLOGY   203

PART FIVE
SPIRITUAL PATHWAYS   273

Introduction
Eddie and Debbie Shapiro

Voices from the Heart came to us as an inspiration from our hearts, as a way to bring greater understanding and compassion to this world. In reaching out to all people to wake up to the choices that we have, this book contains messages from those individuals striving to create a world that is sane. From the beginning, *Voices* took on a life of its own. Almost all of the pieces are from original interviews, and as we spoke with each contributor or gathered their words together, their voices began to weave a tapestry with an ever-deepening message that each one of us can make a difference. This book is a call to wake up to the intrinsic beauty within us and around us, to find the nurturing, caring, and kinder places within ourselves.

Emerging from three years in the Auschwitz concentration camp, psychiatrist Victor Frankl said that with the imprisonment and destruction of his family, he had been left with only "the last of the human freedoms, to choose one's attitude in any given set of circumstances, to choose one's own way." That is the choice that each one of us has—a choice of how we live our lives, how we care for each other, and how we treat our planet. As we move into the new millennium, we have to activate that choice to bring about the changes that are so needed. As we open to transformation within ourselves, so society also transforms; every change that each individual makes creates a chain reaction that is of benefit to all.

We are each so similar. Beneath the color of our skin lie the same organs, the same blood and tissue; we breathe the same air. We are so similar, yet the differences in our minds become vast and create a separation, ignorance, and hatred that blind us to who we truly are.

With so much misunderstanding, life can appear hopeless. Greed, hatred, and delusion are forces that deaden the spirit. The challenges we are confronted with are numerous: ecological and environmental systems are proving to be fragile if not beyond repair; the population is rapidly reaching capacity. But instead of focusing on the problems, we must start living the solutions. To walk fearlessly in the world takes great courage.

Each of us has a voice that longs to speak from the depths of our hearts. It is a yearning for sanity and mercy, for respect and dignity, not just for ourselves but for all beings; it is our longing to feel a connected part of the whole. The voices included here are just examples of the beauty that it is possible to realize within ourselves. This book is dedicated to lifting us out of our fear and into the knowledge that all things are possible, but ultimately we are the only ones who can do this. We have a chance to deepen our commitment to our sanity and dignity and to activate a more meaningful purpose to life. In this way compassion will flourish.

Part 1 explores what we can do individually, for each voice does count; we are all needed. We have different roles to play, like the various instruments that make up an orchestra, but each one is essential for the full symphony. We are all responsible for the whole, as seen in the words of the Dalai Lama, who urges us to open our hearts to universal altruism, and Robert Thurman, who takes us beyond our limited sense of ourselves to recognizing the bigger picture. It is time to go beyond the separatism that divides spirituality from politics, art, education, culture, or the rest of our lives and to live with greater awareness of the whole.

Part 2 shows us how remarkable the effect of just one person's work can be, in contributions from Millard Fuller, who is responsible for thousands of people now having a decent place to live; Dr. A. T. Ariyaratne, who has transformed Sri Lanka through bringing together the villagers and creating community; to John Bird, who went from being a small-time thief to being a Communist to creating a means for the homeless to rebuild their lives. These and others are people whose level of commitment motivates them beyond any hindrances that might appear. Such people inspire us to realize that we should never feel helpless or hopeless, for change is always possible. Each and every one of us has the capacity for transformation by opening our heart. This is seen so clearly in the work with prisoners of both Cathrine Sneed and Bo Lozoff, who recognize that inside each of us is a heart longing to be free.

This book is also about healing the wounds of separation that keep us in fear and loneliness so that compassion and mercy become our means of communication. This is seen so poignantly in Sheila Cassidy's contribution in Part 3, in which she shares her experiences of torture in Chile. The suffering that is both within and around us demands our recognition and mercy. From our own pain grow the awareness and generosity of heart to embrace others in pain, as seen in Dean Ornish's personal journey and the work of Rachel Naomi Remen with cancer patients. As Stephen Levine so clearly shares with us, the pain of another is also our pain; there is no difference.

Part 4 reminds us how altruism can be practiced in every part of our lives, such as in business and the care of our environment. There are solutions to be found; there are answers to our fears, as both Paul Hawken and Helena Norberg-Hodge show us. We are not powerless or helpless in the face of destruction; we do have ways we can implement now to practice greater responsibility to our world. Muhammad Yunus explains how so little can help so many through the use of microcredit to bring dignity of purpose to millions of the poorest, while Mikhail Gorbachev, who transformed the U.S.S.R., reminds us of the need for simplicity and humility through the memory of his peasant upbringing.

Now is the time to communicate and listen to each other, to stop the wars within, and to find ways to develop compassion, forgiveness, and cooperation in every aspect of our lives, as Archbishop Desmond Tutu has so clearly demonstrated in South Africa. Part 5 focuses on qualities of ego and freedom, so that we may discover the open heart and the guru—the true teacher—within ourselves, as seen in the contributions from both Swami Satchidananda and Ram Dass. Spirituality is not the same thing to all people; by finding our own means of worship and ritual, we awaken to a world of beauty and grace.

Working with the contributors to this book was a time of great heart opening for ourselves as editors. Many times tears filled our eyes; many times we wondered with awe at the power of the human spirit. And many times we had to acknowledge the countless voices that are not in this book yet are quietly working for the benefit of all others. In honor of all these voices, both heard and unheard, proceeds from this book will be donated to charities around the world.

May all beings be free to realize the dreams that reside in their hearts. May all beings be free from suffering.

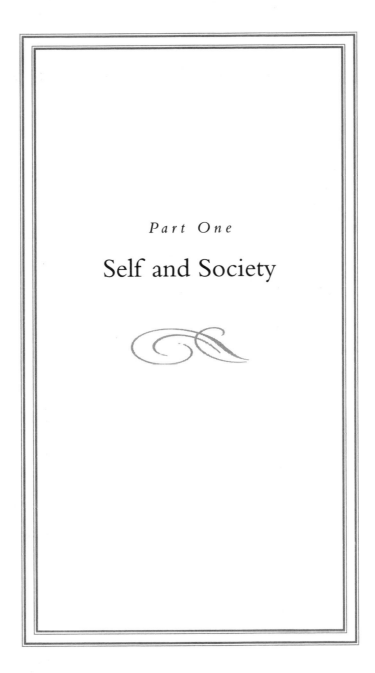

Part One

Self and Society

H. H. The Dalai Lama

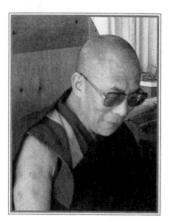

Witnessing profound suffering among his people while living in exile in India since the Chinese invasion of Tibet, the Dalai Lama has become an icon of compassion and forgiveness. As both spiritual and temporal leader of Tibet, his message of universal responsibility has reached millions worldwide. "If we are to protect this home of ours," he says, "each of us needs to experience a vivid sense of universal altruism."

Compassion and Universal Responsibility

In Tibet we say that many illnesses can be cured by the one medicine of love and compassion. These qualities are the ultimate source of human happiness, and our need for them lies at the very core of our being. Unfortunately, love and compassion have been omitted from too many spheres of social interaction for too long. Usually confined to family and home, their practice in public life is considered impractical, even naive. This is tragic. In my view, the practice of compassion is not just a symptom of unrealistic idealism but the most effective way to pursue the best interests of others as well as our own.

The foundation for the development of good relations with one another is altruism, compassion, and forgiveness. Forgiveness is the most effective way of dealing with arguments; altruism and forgiveness bring humanity together so that no conflict, however serious, will go beyond the bounds of what is truly human. A mind committed to compassion is like an overflowing reservoir—a constant source of energy, determination, and kindness. Or this mind can be likened to a seed; when cultivated, it gives rise to many other qualities, such as tolerance, inner strength, and the confidence to overcome fear and insecurity. The compassionate mind is also like an elixir: it is capable of transforming bad situations into beneficial ones. Therefore, we should not limit our expressions of love and compassion to our family and friends. Nor is compassion only the responsibility of clergy or health-care or social workers. It is the necessary business of every part of the human community.

One great question underlies our experience, whether we think about it consciously or not: What is the purpose of life? I believe that the purpose of life is to be happy. From the moment of birth, every human being wants happiness and does not want to suffer. From the very core of our being we simply desire contentment. I don't know whether the universe, with its countless galaxies, stars, and planets, has a deeper meaning, but at the very least it is clear that we humans who live on this Earth face the task of making a happy life for ourselves. Therefore, it is important to discover what will bring about the greatest degree of happiness.

For a start, it is possible to divide every kind of happiness and suffering into two main categories: mental and physical. Of the two, it is the mind that exerts the greatest influence on most of us. Unless we are either gravely ill or deprived of basic necessities, our physical condition plays a secondary role in life. If the body is content, we virtually ignore it. The mind, however, registers every event, no matter how small. Hence we should devote our most serious efforts to bringing about mental peace. From my own limited experience, I have found that the greatest degree of inner tranquility comes from the development of love and compassion.

The more we care for the happiness of others, the greater our own sense of well-being becomes. Cultivating a close, warmhearted feeling for others automatically puts the mind at ease. This helps remove whatever fears or insecurities we may have and gives us the strength to cope with any obstacles we encounter. It is the ultimate source of success in life.

As long as we live in this world, we are bound to encounter problems. If, at such times, we lose hope and become discouraged, we diminish our ability to face difficulties. If, on the other hand, we remember that it is not just ourselves but everyone who has to undergo suffering, this more realistic perspective will increase our determination and capacity to overcome troubles. Indeed, with this attitude, each new obstacle can be seen as yet another valuable opportunity to improve our mind. Thus we can strive gradually to become more compassionate, by developing both genuine sympathy for others' suffering and the will to help remove their pain. As a result, our own serenity and inner strength will increase.

Ultimately, the reason why love and compassion bring greatest happiness is simply that from the core of our nature these are deeply appreciated. The need for love lies at the very foundation of human existence. It results from the profound interdependence we all share with one another. However capable and skillful an individual may be, left alone, he or she will not survive. However vigorous and independent we may feel during the most prosperous periods of life, when we are sick, very young, or very old, we must depend on the support of others.

Interdependence, of course, is a fundamental law of nature. Not only higher forms of life but also many of the smallest insects are social beings. The insects, without any religion or law, survive by mutual cooperation based on an innate recognition of their interconnectedness. The laws of nature dictate that bees, for instance, work together in order to survive. As a result, they possess an instinctive sense of social responsibility. They have no constitution, laws, police, religion, or moral training, but because of their nature, they labor faithfully together on a basis of mutual cooperation. Human beings, on the other hand, have constitutions, vast legal systems, and police forces; we also have religion, remarkable intelligence, and a heart with a great capacity to love. But despite our many extraordinary qualities, in practice we lack a sense of responsibility toward our fellow humans. In some ways I feel we are poorer than the bees.

For instance, millions of people live together in large cities all over the world, but despite this proximity, many are lonely. Some do not have even one human being with whom to share their deepest feelings, and they live in a state of perpetual agitation. Some years ago I met some scientists in the United States who said that the rate of mental illness in their country was quite high—around 12 percent of the population. It became clear during our discussion that the main cause of the depression was not a lack of material necessities but a deprivation of the affection of others. This is very sad. Humans are not solitary animals that associate only in order to mate. If we were, why would we build such large cities and towns?

I believe that despite the rapid advances made by civilization in this century, the most immediate cause of our present dilemma is our undue emphasis on material development alone. We have become so engrossed in its pursuit that, without even knowing it, we have neglected to foster the most basic human needs of love, kindness, cooperation, and caring. But the development of human society is based entirely on people helping each other. Once we have lost the essential humanity that is our foundation, what is the point of pursuing only material improvement?

To me it is clear: a genuine sense of responsibility can result only if we develop compassion. It is because our own human existence is so dependent on the help of others that our need for love lies at the very foundation of our existence. Therefore we need to develop a genuine sense of responsibility and a sincere concern for the welfare of others. I believe that no one is born free from the need for love. And this demonstrates that, although some modern schools of thought seek to do so, human beings cannot be defined as solely physical. No material object, however beautiful or valuable, can make us feel loved, because our deeper identity and true character lie in the subjective nature of the mind.

However, it is also true that we all have an innate self-centeredness that inhibits our love for others. So, since we desire the true happiness that is brought about only by a calm mind and since such peace of mind is brought about only by a compassionate attitude, how can we develop this? Obviously, it is not enough for us simply to think about how nice compassion is! We need to make a concerted effort to develop it; we must use all the events of our daily lives to transform our thoughts and behavior.

First of all, we must be clear about what we mean by compassion. Many forms of compassionate feeling are mixed with desire and attachment. True compassion is not just an emotional response but a firm commitment founded on reason. Therefore, a truly compassionate attitude toward others does not change even if they behave negatively toward us. Of course, developing this kind of compassion is not at all easy.

Whether people are beautiful and friendly, or unattractive and disruptive, ultimately they are human beings, just like ourselves. Like us, they want happiness and do not want suffering. Furthermore, their right to overcome suffering and be happy is equal to our own. Now, when we recognize that all beings are equal in both their desire for happiness and their right to obtain it, we automatically feel empathy for and closeness to them. Through accustoming our minds to this sense of universal altruism, we develop a feeling of responsibility for others: the wish to help them actively overcome their problems. Nor is this wish selective; it applies equally to all. As long as they are human beings experiencing pleasure and pain just as we do, there is no logical basis to discriminate between them or to alter our concern for them if they behave negatively.

Let me emphasize that it is within our power, given patience and time, to develop this kind of compassion. Of course, our self-centeredness, our distinctive attachment to the feeling of an independent, self-existent "I," works fundamentally to inhibit our compassion. Indeed, true compassion can be experienced only when this type of self-grasping is eliminated. But this does not mean that we cannot start and make progress now.

I must emphasize again that merely thinking that compassion and reason and patience are good will not be enough to develop them. We must wait for difficulties to arise and then attempt to practice them. And who creates such opportunities? Not our friends, of course, but our enemies. They are the ones who give us the most trouble. So if we wish to learn, we should consider our enemies to be our best teachers. For a person who cherishes compassion and love, the practice of tolerance is essential, and for that, an enemy is indispensable. So we should feel grateful to our enemies, for it is they who can best help us develop a tranquil mind.

Because we all share an identical need for love, it is possible to feel that anybody we meet, in whatever circumstances, is a brother or sister. No matter how new the face or how different the dress and behavior, there is no significant division between us and other people. It is foolish to dwell on external differences, because our basic natures are the same. I try to treat whomever I meet as an old friend. This gives me a genuine feeling of happiness. It is the practice of compassion.

Ultimately, humanity is one and this small planet is our only home. If we are to protect this home of ours, each of us needs to experience a vivid sense of universal altruism. It is only this feeling that can remove the self-centered motives that cause people to deceive and misuse one another. If we have a sincere and open heart, we naturally feel self-worth and confidence, and there is no need to be fearful of others. The key to a happier world is the growth of compassion. We do not need to become religious, nor do we need to believe in an ideology. All that is necessary is for each of us to develop our good human qualities.

I believe that to meet the challenge of our times, human beings will have to develop a greater sense of universal responsibility. We must all learn to work not just for our own self, family, or nation but for the benefit of all humankind. Universal responsibility is the key to human survival. It is the best foundation for world peace, the equitable use of natural resources, and through concern for future generations, the proper care of the environment.

Marianne Williamson

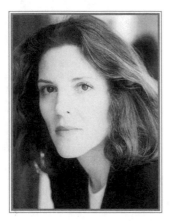

Through her work as an inspirational speaker and writer, Marianne Williamson has made the Course in Miracles accessible to people worldwide. Here she emphasizes the need for us all to stop focusing so much on ourselves and to put into practice the truth we already know. "There is no metaphysical or spiritual justification for turning our eyes away from human suffering."

Time to Stop Hiding

The heart has been relegated to a back seat in world affairs, and the head, when it lacks the counsel of the heart, leads us in dangerous directions. Western civilization now places concern for the market before concern for principle, conscience, and the safety of our children to an extremely dangerous degree.

Our spiritual purpose is to bind the Earth to heaven—to achieve within ourselves and within our worldly structures emanations of pure love. We can harness the all-powerful alchemy of love itself to remove all fear and violence from the Earth.

In a way it is very simple. Every time we see a child who is happy, loved, well cared for, and well educated, every time we experience an environment in which people are creative and happy, their talents and abilities are put to good use, and they live harmoniously with the world around them—that's the blessing; that's it! And that reality is possible for every man, woman, and child on this Earth. If it is present anywhere, it can be present everywhere. Once enough of us hold that vision and work in whichever way we can toward the day of its manifestation, we will achieve an awesome feat.

The great work of our time is the great work of every time, which is to make higher Truth a universal reality. What makes this time different is that we no longer have the luxury of choice; we will evolve to a higher plane of spiritual awareness, or we will all be engulfed in the flames of a world that is bound to go down.

Saying that love will heal us is easy enough to do. Actually achieving the level of profound forgiveness that will release that love is a much more difficult task. We won't be able to do it alone. We will need celestial help to lift us out of our unconscious addiction to the ways of a guilt-ridden world. It is easy to forgive people when we like who they are and particularly when we like what they do. But the forgiveness that will ultimately free this world lies in our capacity to love even those whom we do not like and to forgive what might seem unforgivable.

From Northern Ireland to Bosnia to the United States' street gangs, entrenched enemies will not become friends by anything as simple as deciding to talk over lunch. Hatred is a powerful foe, so powerful that nothing short of God's love can undo it. That is our task: to harness God's love for the purposes of healing not only our own hearts but our streets' and nations' as well.

Both Mahatma Gandhi and Martin Luther King, Jr., applied the principles of nonviolence to the political and social issues of their time, claiming that "soul force is greater than brute force." As Dr. King said, "We have a power in our hearts more powerful than bullets." The moral challenge of our times is to use and release that power.

Nonviolence is not something we can agendize, organize, or strategize. It reflects an inward turning, a melting of the heart which alone melts the walls outside us. It is a particularly potent concept when applied to a democracy, because what goes on within the democratic citizen becomes, when expressed, the fuel for society's engine.

The word *politics* stems from an ancient Greek root that means "of the state and citizen." What goes on inside the citizen—our anger and despair as well as our hopes and our capacity to forgive—all carries political significance. Our whole selves must be brought to bear on the effort to transform human civilization. As Dr. King said, we must have "tough minds and tender hearts." Most people I know tend to have one or the other: some who have the toughest minds often lack tender hearts, whereas some of the most open hearted among us often lack intellectual acumen. Fuzzy thinking is just one step above not thinking. We must find the lion as well as the lamb within us; it is in their lying down together that we rise to our divine potential.

The political activist without spiritual wisdom is blind, but the spiritual activist without political understanding is ineffective. I believe that there are millions of people ready to take the next step toward the intersection of our political and spiritual goals—to try, as did Gandhi and King before us, to lift the love in our hearts to a level of a large-scale social force for the good.

First, we must be willing to open our eyes, to repudiate our layers of thick denial regarding the disparate state of so much of humanity. There is no metaphysical or spiritual justification for turning our eyes away from human suffering. We cannot bring forth resurrection in an environment in which we have denied the crucifixion. The spiritual seeker is often vulnerable to the "I care therefore I don't have to do anything" syndrome. But, quite simply, just caring is not enough. In fact, it is an interesting moral question of our generation: If you care about those in need and you do nothing to help them, do you get more points in heaven or fewer?

Self-awareness is a critically important thing, but we must always be aware of the line past which self-awareness becomes self-preoccupation. The spiritual seeker must be on guard against the narcissism and self-indulgence that can far too easily and insidiously plague us as we set out on the inward-turning path. I have no interest in coddling those who already have the tools with which to deal with their issues. A generation of Americans that has gotten in touch with its pain from childhood more than any other generation on record now presides over a scandalous neglect of our nation's children.

Very critical issues are unfolding in the world around us, and they are much bigger than any one particular person's neuroses. Spirituality should not be a form of escapism from the horrors and the dangers of the world; it should be a context for their transformation. And enough of us are ready now to take on the job; we know the principles, we have read the same books, and we have listened to the same tapes. A critical mass of us are no longer seekers but pilgrims. The seeker doesn't know yet what the path is, whereas the pilgrim does know the path but is dealing with a daily resistance to walking it. It is the pilgrims among us who must make the journey on behalf of the entire world.

The transformation of the world will be brought about not through a lateral but through a vertical effort: it is not only what we do but who we now choose to become that will determine the future of Earth. I am optimistic because we have choice; the mass intention to change, to awaken from our spiritual slumber, will bring about miraculous results. But God knows how potent are the lullabies that would have us remain asleep through the problems. There is so much stress, so many grown-up toys to buy, so much television to put our minds to sleep, so many games we are seemingly addicted to playing. And most of the suffering among us is on the other side of town. These are very easy times to sleep through. However, whatever we choose will be visited on our children. God help them if we do not wake up.

We live in a very critical moment, and each one among us is being asked by God to be a conduit for His work. We don't have to worry how God will transmit the instructions to us; if we are humble enough and willing enough, He will find a way. If we are willing to forgive and bless each other, if we seriously pray and meditate and practice the ways of devotion, if we follow our hearts whenever we feel there is a chance for us to serve an unfolding good, then we will contribute to a great wave of change. A shift of historic proportions is already under way as humanity makes the effort to evolve from an inner state of war to an outer state of peace. We are all just servants of a master plan. All we have to do is simply do what we can, then give praise and give thanks. The rest will follow.

Christopher Titmuss

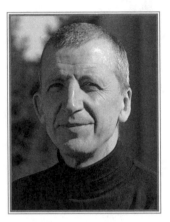

From being a Buddhist monk to standing as a Green Party candidate, Christopher Titmuss views teaching meditation and political and social action with the same eyes. In the following pages he explores their mutual territory and interconnectedness. "I do not consider myself to be a meditation teacher sometimes and a social activist at other times," he says. "I just focus on making a contribution to liberation through the resolution of the problems of humanity."

Awareness: Springboard
for Meditation and Politics

I lead retreats in insight meditation and I have twice stood for Parliament for the Green Party. Teaching meditation and engaging in political action can appear to be worlds apart, but in fact they are the same thing; both authentic meditation and authentic political awareness challenge the ego. I do not consider myself a social activist; liberation of all beings is my only interest, and I believe liberation concerns every area of life from the inner to the political. True meditation and social action spring from an awareness and understanding of liberation that embraces inner and outer circumstances equally.

In Israel I met a Palestinian hero figure who is confronting the Israeli building program in East Jerusalem. He sits on the hill opposite where they are building, under a large, black canopy with Palestinian flags, as a symbol of protest. Many people go to visit him. The Israelis have cleared the forest and they are building, but he stays there, opposing. Looking at the building site, he said to me, "What's with meditation, when we have all this?" I answered, "First there is vision. Then there is awareness, which brings action. Meditation is there to keep the mind absolutely steady, so it doesn't fall into violence, aggression, and loss of vision." I regard meditation as a resource for stability, clarity, insight, and opening of the heart; it enables vision to stay focused as awareness brings its own action.

I can't imagine meditation separate from concern for the world. However, there is a difference between criticism and negativity, between constructive engagement and the dualism of "us and them." We do not need to regard one as the cause for the other. I do not believe that the self creates its own problems or that other people create our problems: problems arise simply because the conditions for them come into being. Nor do I believe that I have an exclusive inner truth or that some people have more of the truth than others. I do not consider myself to be a meditation teacher sometimes and a social activist at other times; I just focus on making a contribution to liberation through the resolution of the problems of humanity. Some problems appear to be located within the individual, and other problems within the structures that society has created for itself. But the mind and the structures remain inseparable from each other.

We need to dispense with the dualism of spirituality and politics, abandon all the associations that we have with these two areas, and look at things afresh. Then we may see that the two are already engaged. It shows itself in every word we say, every breath we take, and every moment of mindfulness. Engagement means a direct, active contribution toward the resolution of the problems of life.

The attitude of nonviolence plays an important role here, in both meditation and politics. The function of nonviolence comes from three specific standpoints. First is moral injunction from which we might be prone to violence or retaliation, but as violence goes against our beliefs or values, we put a restraining order on our actions so as to maintain our commitment to nonviolence in the deeper sense.

Second is the depth of insight and realization that cannot give support to capital punishment or to inflicting violence intentionally on other human beings. At this point nonviolence has gone beyond an act of will and has entered into a way of understanding.

Third is the approach of nonviolence as a useful and effective strategy. Killing and harming are gross tactics to deal with social, political, and economic problems. Violence, including throwing stones, firing bullets, laying land mines, or planting bombs, creates fear and mistrust. Strikes, demonstrations, noncooperation, negotiation, leaflets, and humor are more effective strategies and generate greater international support.

I was a monk with Venerable Maha Ghosananda, who exemplifies constructive nonviolence. He is Cambodian. He had seventeen relatives and all were murdered during the mid-1970s. Venerable Ghosananda left the monastery to work in the refugee camps of the Cambodians in Thailand. When the doors reopened, he went back to his country. Every May he walks through Cambodia to bring peace and justice. He went to the soldiers and said to them, "Lay down your rifles and kill the hate inside yourselves." He went to the parents of the soldiers and told them to tell their sons to lay down their rifles and kill the hate inside themselves. He went to the children of the soldiers and told them to tell their fathers. And so on. He has been nominated for the Nobel Peace Prize four times. We stood together on the steps of Capitol Hill in a UN-sponsored demonstration. Venerable Ghosananda told the media, "The land mines in the ground come from the land mines in our minds. We must uproot both."

I believe it is so important that the voices of constructive engagement take priority, or, as a former Palestinian freedom fighter told me, we must exchange words instead of bullets. We must keep faith with the strategies and approaches of constructive protest and engagement, no matter how difficult particular situations appear to be.

Three years ago I was asked to go to the West Bank and to take a select number of Israelis to spend three days there in Palestinian homes. This served as a springboard to other extended visits and to forming an organization, Face to Face. It aims to sustain contact with

Palestinians, to lower the degree of fear, mistrust, and anger as a contribution to understanding. On a recent trip the Israeli authorities had stopped entrance into the West Bank, so I went alone to the control point and walked across. I spent the day with my Palestinian friends and then brought back the report of what I had heard and seen to the Face to Face group. At that time there was a tremendous loss of faith in the peace process, and the result was Hamas terrorist bomb attacks. The people were despairing.

My work is dealing with the mutual understanding of each other and the tightness of identification of being an Israeli or a Palestinian. Meditation is not the reference point; rather it is communication and language. People must meet and get to know each other so that they see the common ground—their shared humanity, suffering, fear, insecurity. Then things start shifting. We all have far more in common than what separates us, and the communication has to be kept going at all cost, no matter how bad it may seem.

There are few things that I feel to be more important than working with anger. Anger harms ourselves as much as others. It is an ineffective way to achieve anything as it simply invites defensiveness or withdrawal from others, reinforcing dualism. There is no usefulness in any form of anger as a way of resolving human conflict. To imagine that we can just be angry toward one particular authority but full of kindness everywhere else is delusion. Any level of anger is unacceptable.

If we are not angry, then where will the energy come from, the adrenalin, that will motivate us to act? In fact, we need only the awareness of suffering; that should be enough to motivate anybody. When motivation is clear, then awareness is there. These two factors are vital, as is practicing loving-kindness meditation and equanimity. If anger is not being resolved inwardly, then we have to associate with those who maintain clear and constructive engagement. We're asking too much of people to be able to resolve their despair alone.

I can't imagine anybody having wisdom or compassion without a community—a sangha—that gives ongoing support.

In 1990, several of us put together a school for about twenty children in Bodh Gaya. It is located in the middle of the state of Bihar, certainly the poorest state of India and maybe of South Asia. The school provides the poorest of the poor with education as a vital stepping-stone to awareness and change. We started off in a very modest way, but the school has now grown to some three hundred children. It is a true sangha, a vibrant community. There are Catholic nuns, Buddhist monks, Hindus, and Muslims all teaching in the school.

Our function as Westerners is to provide the financial resources to run the school and to ensure that the teachers are genuinely committed to interreligious awareness. We are not becoming colonial educationalists. In a talk to both Westerners and Asians there, Sister Jesse, a much-loved person, said it is not enough just to give money. We must make sacrifices and be prepared to offer something other than money. She said, "If you only have money to give, then you may as well throw it into the Bay of Bengal!" It was a dramatic statement. She was asking us to really extend ourselves.

I suspect that as we move into the new millennium, there will be a period of soul-searching among the affluent nations about their relationships to each other and to the rest of the world. Selfishness is the virus that pervades the human species. It destroys lives, communities, the welfare of societies, and Earth itself. Five years ago I had a meeting with one of my teachers, Achaan Buddhadasa. He spoke at length to me about selfishness. He commented rather wryly, "We won't destroy this world through ignorance but through being too clever. We have become too clever for our own good and too clever for everybody else's good." We must ask ourselves again and again what our priorities are. Is our daily life an honest statement of what matters? If not, we are wasting our existence on the trivial and immaterial. Our daily life states our values. There is no other criteria; we live by what we believe.

What do so many of the world's great heroes have in common? Meditation. They know the importance of the depths of meditation and awareness to contribute to loving-kindness. When we see the truth of who we are, then we know humanity is one, not fragmented. This vision influences our feelings, thoughts, and actions. We know that self and others are not separate. The war within has stopped.

Winona LaDuke

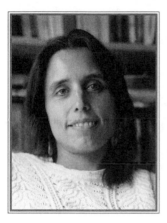

Winona LaDuke is a Native American and indigenous people's rights activist, as well as a campaigner for environmental issues. In her piece she shares the role of women in indigenous nations and applauds a few of the many women who have withstood massive political opposition. "The courage of those women is the courage that carries us forward."

Indigenous Women

I am an Anishinabe, which means "people." We are called Chippewa in the United States and Ojibwe in Canada. There are about seven hundred native communities in North America today: indigenous peoples who define themselves according to who they are in their own destiny, in their own memory, in their own history. They are peoples who share a common language, territory, and governing and economic institutions. It is said that on a worldwide scale there are five thousand nations of indigenous people. Yet, on a worldwide scale, most decisions are not made by nations. They are made by states. And most decision-making states have only been in existence for the past two hundred years, some of them only since World War II.

On our 4 percent of North American land we have two-thirds of the nation's uranium resources, one-third of all low-sulphur strippable coal resources, the single largest hydroelectric project, and vast oil and gas reserves, yet the systematic dispossession of our land has made us the poorest people in this country. Elsewhere in the world we are peoples on the brink of economic and ecological disaster. Seventy percent of the wars in the world involve indigenous peoples, usually wars between nations and states trying to annex the land. Almost all nuclear testing that has occurred in the world has occurred either on the land or in the water of indigenous peoples. In the Boreal rain forests of Canada 50 percent of all reservation land is forested, but the rate of clear-cutting is one acre every eleven seconds. In Brazil the rate is one acre every nine seconds. Today, the Western Shoshone Nation is the most bombed nation on earth, with over seven hundred nuclear tests conducted on the Shoshone land. These are issues about our collective ability to determine our destiny.

We see the issues of the indigenous woman as the issues of all peoples; native women are seen as the backbones of our nations. There is a Cheyenne saying that "a nation is not defeated until the hearts of its women are on the ground." In our own Ojibwe stories, original woman came and stood on the shell of a turtle after the great flood. She asked the animals to help her form the earth. Bear said, "I can help you. I am a very good swimmer. I will go down to the bottom of the water and I will get some earth." But Bear could not do it; he did not have the strength. Then Otter came and said, "I am a better swimmer than Bear. I will swim down to the bottom and I will get the earth." So Otter tried, but he also failed. Each animal tried and failed in succession, until finally Muskrat, the smallest and most pitiful of the animals, said, "I will try." And they all laughed and scoffed at Muskrat, but Muskrat went all the way down to the bottom of the ocean and grabbed a tiny piece of earth. By the time he got back to the surface he was dead, but in his little fist there was a piece of earth. That is the story of how the earth got formed and how it was woman who arranged the forming.

It is said that the U.S. form of democracy was founded on the concepts of the Iroquois confederacy, the idea of the division between different branches of government and of representational democracy. But the founding fathers missed a very essential point. In the Iroquois six-nation confederacy, the clan mothers had the right to appoint and depose chiefs; mothers of those slain in battle held sway over prisoners and could intervene in the conduct of war. However, the role of women was not cast so favorably in the eyes of the Europeans. The concept of patriarchy came from Europe, so the colonists looked at native communities through patriarchal eyes; they did not recognize the status of native women as there was not that same understanding in their own societies. The founding fathers did not even give women the right to vote.

When there were treaties to be signed in the United States or Canada, the signatories were men because the colonists assumed that men had the greater authority. They disregarded women as authority figures, as well as property holders. Yet in my community, all property associated with a house belongs to the woman, not the man. When there is a separation between a couple, the woman puts the man's things outside the house. And that is true in most indigenous communities: the man owns the things that are his, but the woman owns the house.

The imagery of native women needs to be remade. This is not unique to native women; it is a struggle that we must all go through in one way or another—the struggle to redefine ourselves and our identity within our own naming, within our own ways. We think of our grandmothers, the women who were before us, about what they stood for and how we are able to do our work now because someone resisted before us. The courage of those women is the courage that carries us forward.

I think of Mary and Carie Dann, Shoshone women who live in Nevada and who won the Right Livelihood Award because they stood against relocation and against the military testing of nuclear weapons on their land. I think of Elizabeth Penashue and Mary Pasteen, two elderly Innu women in northern Labrador. They have been fighting a military base in Goose Bay where much of Europe tests its military. They have low-level flying up there. Mary and Elizabeth go and stand on the runway and watch fifty-ton fighter jets take off over their heads and fly just above the treetops. They resist this because low-level flying destroys their way of life, destroys their hunting territory, destroys them as people.

I think of women from Chiapas in Mexico who live in a militarized zone. They wear ski masks because if their faces are seen when they leave the village, they will probably be killed by the military. I sat with four women who were my age, one of whom was nursing a small child, and asked them why they took up arms. The mother said to me, "We are tired of living like animals. We are tired of having our dignity stripped from us. We are tired of not being able to make a living from our land, and we are tired of the military. So we took up arms because we wanted a better life. We wanted to be treated like human beings." I looked at this woman and all I could think of was that the United States gave $250 million of military aid to that country in 1996—a country like Mexico with no known enemies. Who is going to invade Mexico? That was all I could think of when I saw her face.

I think of Margaret Palmer, who has been arrested many times on the Columbia River for fishing. If you are an Indian person in the Northwest, you can go to jail for fishing, because fishing appears to have become the exclusive right of factory trawlers. But Margaret Palmer goes to her accustomed fishing place on the Columbia River and stands on a fishing scaffold, which is a rickety set of boards that go out over the river rushing by about thirty feet below. She goes way out there on this plank, with a rope around her waist that ties her to the shore and with a dip net, and gets fish. That is what you get arrested for if you are an Indian person on the Columbia River. But she has stood against the state of Washington and the state of Oregon, and she has stood against the federal government. Now she also fights a luxury home development that is seeking to surround her in a form of "ecotourism" because windsurfing seems to be very popular where she happens to fish. She said, "I will not come to this place, where the fish have given up their spirits to my ancestors and me. I will not fish in the shadow of a luxury home development. I will not fish in the shadow of their swimming pools."

I think of Levina White, a nearly blind Haider woman from the Northwest Coast, who talks about reclaiming who you are. She said, "I am speaking to you on behalf of the 'wildlife,' as you call it. Everything you call wild we call natural. And when you call it wild, that means you want to tame it." We have to start changing our wording. We talk about power and empowerment, but let us talk about responsibility. We talk about management of the environment, but perhaps we should be managing mankind, not the environment.

At the U.N. conference on the status of women in Beijing, China, I was interested in why women, from very remote villages or small island states, who had very little money, would struggle to get to a U.N. conference. What did they hope to accomplish? Susannah Ounei is a Kanake woman, from what the French call New Caledonia in the Pacific. She said, "It started in 1853 when the French thought they had discovered savages, the lost race of Melanesia. They found our beautiful islands, they saw nickel, gold, copper, and magnesium, and they killed over two hundred thousand of our people for the land. For the past decade the Kanakes have been in an armed struggle against the French. Now the French have scheduled a referendum for the end of the century, but meantime they are transplanting French citizens to New Caledonia so that they can weight the referendum. So while a few years ago the Kanakes were the majority of the population, today they are 43 percent in their own country."

Susannah says, "Give us back our dignity, values, and land. That is what we want." She watches the French detonate an atomic bomb near French Melanesia in the Pacific and says, "If it is so safe, why do they not test it in Versailles?" I ask her why she is at the conference and she says, "Because Mrs. Chirac is here. She does not come to see me on my island, so I come here to see her."

Mililani Trask, head of state of the traditional Hawaiian government, is a woman who has fought the federal government's right to Hawaii. The queen of Hawaii was overthrown in 1893, and then the islands were annexed by the United States in 1959. But, under U.S. law, native Hawaiians do not have the same rights as other American citizens. There are three classes of citizens in the United States who do not have the right to go into federal court: retarded individuals, minors, and native Hawaiians. The native Hawaiians said, "We are a nation, and we are reorganizing and restructuring our form of government." The U.S. government said, "You cannot do that." Mililani Trask said, "You just watch." She organized twenty-two thousand Hawaiians to form the beginning of a new nation of Hawaii. She said, "We are going to sign a treaty between the native Hawaiians and the Macah Indians." The federal government said, "You cannot sign a treaty. We are the only people who can approve treaties." She said, "You just watch. Nations make treaties and we are a nation of people. We will make a treaty." And they signed it.

Mililani Trask was at the U.N. conference because, as she said, "I live on a small island, but my small place is part of the big pool that is the world. There are twenty-seven species of bird that are on the endangered species list on my island. And all twenty-seven of those species nest in a place called the Arctic National Wildlife Refuge, in the north of the United States, a place that the Congress wants to open for oil development. Those species will not be protected unless I go to the international arena."

So what can we learn from these women and their struggles? Maybe we can take courage from their courage. Women who struggle in the face of great adversaries, who struggle in meager circumstances with far less resources than ourselves, but women who know the difference between being poor and being powerless. Many indigenous people know that they are repressed, but they do not feel powerless. Perhaps we can learn that each of us has the right to define who we are and that we do not have to relinquish that right to anyone else. I do not relinquish my right of definition to a transnational corporation or to the government. Our right of self-definition is something that we hold in our hearts.

Perhaps we can also learn from these women about the absence of recourse under the law. There is something fundamentally wrong with a law that allows what France did in the Pacific. The founding fathers always believed that we should be able to drink the water and breathe the air. But now Dow Chemical, Monsanto, British Petroleum, and others have made it difficult to be sure that we can drink the water or breathe the air. The question is, what right does a private interest have to affect a common property, not only for this generation but for the seventh generation to come?

One day I was testifying on a resolution at an Exxon stockholders meeting in Chicago. The shareholders' resolution was on Exxon's nuclear holdings, and some antinuclear activists got up and talked about why Exxon should divest itself of this. The shareholders just looked at them and then went on with their business. Then these nuns stood up. Nuns are very good at stockholders' meetings. They said they wanted Exxon to divest its South African holdings. And everybody listened to the nuns and held their heads down because they were all ashamed of their behavior as stockholders and as a corporation. Then I stood up and talked about Exxon's uranium holdings on the Navajo reservation, and they looked at me like I was from outer space.

Then this Maryknoll priest stood up, Father Roy Bourgeois. He spends most of his time challenging the U.S. military in third world countries. Father Roy went to the microphone and said, "I don't have a resolution; I have a question. I have been living in Latin America for the past ten years, and the people there want to know if there is a direct relationship between their poverty and your wealth." And that is all he said. We can talk about human rights in any country in the world, but until we deal with levels of materialism in first world countries it will be meaningless to talk about human rights.

As a woman I consider all these issues to be my issues. I think about why it is I am more concerned about the amount of sugar in my son's breakfast cereal than I am about the amount of mercury or PCBs in his tissues. These are issues about the meaningful definition of our destiny. This is the challenge we collectively face, a challenge that will determine our future. I believe not only that we have the right and the responsibility to undertake this but that with our abilities, our knowledge, and the resource of the wellspring we have inside us, we have the ability to meet it.

Yoko Ono

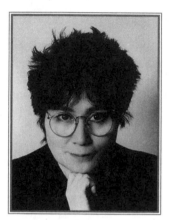

Yoko Ono is a poet, musician, and artist whose paintings grace galleries worldwide. In the following poem she describes how we can transform our weaknesses into strengths.

Bless you for your anger,
For it is a sign of rising energy.
Direct not to your family, waste not on your enemy.
Transform the energy to versatility
And it will bring you prosperity.

Bless you for your sorrow,
For it is a sign of vulnerability.
Share not with your family, direct not to yourself.
Transform the energy to sympathy
And it will bring you love.

Bless you for your greed,
For it is a sign of great capacity.
Direct not to your family, direct not to the world.
Transform the energy to giving.
Give as much as you wish to take
And you will receive satisfaction.

Bless you for your jealousy,
For it is a sign of empathy.

Direct not to your family, direct not to your friends.
Transform the energy to admiration
And what you admire
Will become part of your life.

Bless you for your fear,
For it is a sign of wisdom.
Do not hold yourself in fear.
Transform the energy to flexibility
And you will be free
From what you fear.

Bless you for your search of direction,
For it is a sign of aspiration.
Transform the energy to receptivity
And the direction will come to you.

Bless you for the times you see evil.
Evil is energy mishandled and it feeds on your support.
Feed not and it will self-destruct.
Shed light and it will cease to be.

Bless you for the times you feel no love.
Open your heart to life anyway
And in time you will find
Love in you.

Bless you, bless you, bless you.
Bless you for what you are.
You are a sea of goodness, a sea of love.
Count your blessings every day, for they are your protection
Which stands between you and what you wish not.

Revelations

Count your curses and they will be a wall
Which stands between you and what you wish.

The world has all that you need,
And you have the power
To attract what you wish.
Wish for health, wish for joy.
Remember you are loved.
I love you!

Robert Thurman

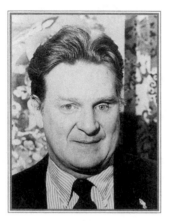

One of Time *magazine's fifty most influential people in 1997, Robert Thurman is widely known for his support of the Dalai Lama and the Tibetan people's campaign for freedom. In this piece he explores his belief that a better world is possible. "Shambhala is the critical mass of people making that shift in their hearts from despair, paranoia, fear, and egotism to openness, vulnerability, and optimism," he says. "If there is going to be some critical moment when there's a massive awakening,, it will only happen because each individual person awakens her or his own heart."*

Shambhala Now

It feels awkward and sad and embarrassing to be leaving the planet in such a tremendous mess for the following generations. Everything is in quite a state. We have the apocalypse looming over us in all kinds of ways. One of the things that keeps me going is that I have a vision that there is a good time ahead, that there is a Shambhala, a New Jerusalem, not just some sort of half-wit fantasy but a real one, around the corner. This will become a reality by people's waking up to the fact that they have the power to make a horrible, destructive age much deeper and worse than this terrible twentieth century has been and that, since they have such a power, they have a responsibility to gain control over themselves to not use that power in such a destructive way.

Human beings have a sort of inbred inferiority complex; we are conditioned to believe that we are weak and inferior and can't really do anything about anything, that either there is some all-powerful God who has handed us this thing or else it's just random permutations of matter, and as there is nothing much we can do about it, we may as well just run for cover. Since there is not enough, there is no need to try to share anything; we just have to make sure we are covered. So we hoard things, and then we create a self-fulfilling prophecy as there isn't enough because we don't share. Trying to defend ourselves, we spend a lot of money on wasteful violence and defense expenditure, and therefore there isn't enough creative expenditure on education and art. And so the planet doesn't work very well. One lesson for humanity to learn from the twentieth century is that there is no limit to human genius. We can blow up the whole planet, we can rip atoms to pieces, we can destroy ourselves totally. We have that power. Once we admit that we have power for good or evil, then we have to take responsibility for whether we use our power for good or evil.

When we look around the world, Shambhala seems further away than ever. We have rulers who seem intelligent and say the right things, but when they get in power, they do a lot of wrong things. They chicken out from speaking the truth; they become self-seeking and self-promoting rather than working for the common good. The good guys get crucified and some bad guy rules. This is the whole world-negating Western view. And if people's natural impulses come out, it'll be bad, so there is original sin. Love is nice; it's fun. A little bit can creep out here and there to have a baby or something and we can worship a savior who resurrects spiritually or a Mary who is assumed into heaven, but love cannot rule on the ground. Anybody who thinks it can is dangerous and crazy.

This is a self-destructive, self-defeating-prophecy type of idea. In Asia they have the experience of good kings who selflessly served the people, who were not addicted to whatever it was and didn't just hide in the palace with some eunuchs but cared about the people and distributed the wealth. This kind of tradition is one of love being the most practical way of living, of love being positive, and therefore of love being what you expect from the government and the rulers because it is most practical. However, in the West, when we are happy, when Romeo is in love with Juliet, we don't expect it to last. We expect something to go wrong or somebody to get murdered. If we ever feel good, we want to run off and hide, because we think somebody is going to come and step on us.

We have to broaden our cultural perspectives from our narrow Western ones and realize that this is our conditioning due to a psychology of scarcity. We have to realize we are a success now, we've made it, we can do what we want with the world. We can wreck it if we want, but we can also run the world effectively and lovingly, and if we do run it that way, it will be cheaper and more practical. But we must stop accepting the idea that we should elect the lesser of two evils, that no government can ever do a decent job, that it's always going to be bad so why bother to vote. Democracy is the skill of people to associate with each other, to be open with each other, and not to suppress the free flow of communication, not to be authoritarian or domineering, not to be afraid of openness. It is people's ability to live in an interconnected way. If we look at our educational system, we don't teach people this. But how do we retrain the individual's heart to be open and to overcome authoritarianism and divisive ideologies like racism, sexism, or religious fanaticism?

I decided long ago that the human mind is capable of understanding everything necessary for life, and it is a question, therefore, of getting the world to take charge of its own fate. Seeing to it that it is a good fate is a matter of getting people to understand their own situation. Saving the world is fundamentally an educational problem. That's why I like the Buddha, because he had great faith in people. At first he didn't know whether people were useless or OK or what. He didn't accept the prevailing wisdom of his time, so he researched deeply and eventually came to the realization that people could understand what was necessary to be understood. They could liberate themselves from suffering, and they could help others to become free from suffering. He saw that it was just a matter of delivering an educational service that they could use, a system that educated the whole being, the heart and every fiber of the body as well as the brain, one that included the intellectual with the emotional, the ethical, and the spiritual.

This is how the Buddha offered a tremendous gift to the planet, not in creating a competing religion but as a service in an educational way. People can use this service while remaining Muslim or Christian or whatever. They don't have to become a member of a religion. The service is to provide methods for looking into our own hearts. You can understand how prejudices are formed on the basis of a misappropriated identity, a wrong attitude about what is a male, a wrong attitude about what is a white or a black or a yellow, a wrong attitude about what it means to be a part of this culture or that religion, a misunderstanding of Mohammed or Jesus or the Buddha, thinking he said you should go out and hate people who don't follow him. Buddhism has this unparalleled methodology—meditational, analytical, and ethical—of how to understand and recondition the human heart.

Democracy can use this methodology; it's a marriage that can turn things around. Everything is so fast today, the political machinery is so powerful, but it will not work if it continues to be operated by people who have no power over themselves. It's good that politicians and leaders have nice ideals; they want to help everybody, they love God, they feel they should be kind to this person or that person. But if they lack methodology they say, "Well, I should love everybody but in fact I dislike most people. I'm irritable, annoyed, proud; I think I'm right and they're wrong; and that's just the way I am." They are not going to be able to follow their ideals and love everybody, because they won't know how. So what is needed is a method through which we can take the way we feel and reshape it. Just as, systematically, I could take a lump of clay and shape it into a beautiful statue, so I can learn to sculpt myself into a new form.

We all have to resculpture ourselves into better beings. And we have to do it systematically, with just as much high tech as we are messing up the world with. Otherwise we're not going to be able to catch up to the momentum of the machinery of uncontrolled material technology operated by people driven by greed, hatred, delusion, pride, and envy. If we don't learn to conquer those five energies and turn them into love, generosity, tolerance, friendliness, and compassion, then we just won't make it. People do not even have to have heard of the Buddha in order to be able to use this concept to open their hearts.

It is no good getting stuck on the idea that everything's so awful, but one day suddenly there's going to be a big ray of light coming out of the heavens and everything's going to change. That's too passive and cynical and dooms too many people. Rather, we should say that the twentieth century has been a total Armageddon already. There were World Wars I and II, and there have been I don't know how many other wars. There have been the internal repressions in the gulags of China and Russia and the famines in Africa; it has been unspeakable. This has been such a devastating century, terribly disastrous and destructive, and it still goes on in Africa and in Tibet; even in the United States we are still taking land from the Native Americans, while the African American and Latino people in our inner cities are in a tremendously embattled state. It's all still going on.

We need to see that the monstrous beast of selfishness and confusion and ignorance begins within our own hearts. Each individual in his or her own life must take responsibility and decide that, "In my heart I'm going to live in a positive way; I'm not going to justify hardening my heart by looking outside and saying it's all so horrible I might as well be horrible to defend myself. I'm going to be positive; in whatever little corner I can I'm going to make a difference."

In the midst of the horror we can find beauty. Shambhala is the critical mass of people making that shift in their hearts from despair, paranoia, fear, and egotism to openness, vulnerability, and optimism. And we can be in Shambhala now, rather than waiting for it to arrive sometime later. If there is going to be a point, some critical moment when lots of people turn round at once and there's a massive awakening, that's good, but it will only happen because each individual person awakens in her or his own heart. One by one, the world will awaken.

We've got to make the goal the means. We can't just create peace by using violence. We have to create peace by being peaceful. And then people will be peaceful. Even harder than being peaceful is being happy, to be cheerful—really cheerful—to be happy and count the blessings. Our human heart thrives on being happy. We are in fact the form of evolution that is most built for pleasure. Scientists go on and on about how the brain is redundant because they can't understand why we need such a big brain just to run out and jab some buffalo with a spear. But that isn't our job. Our job may be to go and caress the buffalo, to be loving and playful and experience pleasure. That's what all the brain is for; it's like a sea anemone that loves to feel pleasure. Our power and greatness come from our ability to see the vision of happiness. Yet we're conditioned to think that if we allow ourselves to be naturally happy, then we're going to be beaten up by an authoritarian parent because we were being too noisy or having too much fun. We're conditioned to feel frightened when we feel happy, and therefore to wall off our sensations of happiness and pleasure and hide them even from ourselves. But we can undo that conditioning. That's what education is about—undoing the conditioning.

All education should do that, in the literal sense of *educare,* to bring out in the person his or her own potential and nature rather than indoctrinate, suppress, or force him or her into a mold. Buddhist education was developed in ancient India, which was the source of all the Yoga and the fabulous stuff they have there; India was like super-California in ancient times. It had a cultural and historical experience of great wealth, plurality, and openness. People were less afraid of the feminine, of connecting to nature and the kindness of the feminine, than they were in the West, where the feminine has been so suppressed in the modern millennia. So many wonderful people in Europe were women who wanted to heal or who had powerful visions, but they were burned. Our social history in the West is just too nasty. We think we're so superior. That's the problem; we don't realize what a tremendously backward bunch of tribes we have been.

While India was overrun first by Muslims and then by Europeans, Tibet stayed untouched up in the mountains. The Tibetan civilization is unique because it did not develop an internal infrastructure of materialism. A very crucial question for the planet is, Why are we not protecting such a civilization? We say we want peace, that we want love and compassion, that we want to be honest and friendly and happy, and then we find a culture where people are mostly like that and we destroy it. We say it's feudal, it's old-fashioned, or it's none of our business.

I work in relation to the efforts of His Holiness the Dalai Lama to try to see to it that the world starts to be honest about Tibet, to see that the political, short-sighted, destructive, and self-serving interests of leaders and multinational corporations are not allowed to destroy that civilization or to deliberately and systematically destroy its people. Governments around the world have been very duplicitous for over a century on this topic; it's not just the Chinese government at all. I feel that since we are, hopefully, dealing with some vestiges of democracy, the thing is to understand the reality of Tibet and know the nature of the Tibetan people, to have the vision of that civilization so that we know what is being lost.

It's a sort of national liberation movement that arises when the heart falls in love with Tibetan civilization, once it realizes what the New Year festival means, what Tibetan medicine or the monastic university system is about, and what Tibetan yogis are. Once people realize that, then there will be a natural energy to save it, which I think will be part of the whole turning of the corner at the end of the twentieth century.

The Tibetan Book of the Dead is one of Tibet's great gifts to the world, because death is the great teacher. Whatever pretensions and confusions and different things people believe as they wind themselves around this and that false piece of security in life, when they get to that unraveling point at death, then they are forced to wake up, at least for that moment. Sadly, it's almost impossible to do it in such a rush, under such pressure. And so they have a hard time dying. But if we think about it beforehand and work at it and we take that healing perspective of the clear light, the openness and letting go of everything that we have to do in death, if we rehearse that and live life under the instruction of death, so to speak, then we will live much more fully, much more openly.

This understanding brings people to being able to cope with this ultimate challenge, death, which is the one thing nobody can cope with. Materialism has made people feel they don't need to bother with death, that all they have to do is buy a good cemetery plot or something, because there's nothing after death. They have come up with this fake excuse, but people know subconsciously that that can't be true because only nothing can be nothing. Somebody can never be nothing.

In the same way we are denying our death, we are denying the reality of our life. If we are not able to recognize death, we cannot know that we are alive, because life cannot have any meaning unless we know the opposite. Life gets its meaning and its freedom from death, because it is death that allows life to flourish. We can live and breathe because we can change; if we didn't have that moment-by-moment release, we'd freeze, like a block of wood. Death is what constantly lubricates our lives, because it is what is changing everything.

Those who refuse to face death are living in some idea of being alive and trying to make things in the world fit with that idea. And since that's impossible, since the world is always more amazing and more elusive than any idea can be, if they try to force themselves into the mold of the idea, then they will be frustrated and will suffer. It doesn't work to try to force the world to fit our own imposed attitudes about it. Only when we learn to go with the world and connect to it and allow it to bring us surprises and be vulnerable to it, can we get beyond suffering.

We have to stop selling ourselves short, stop selling out for less than we can be, for less than we can have, for less than we can give. We don't have to accept the authorities' curtailment of our capability. But let's be intelligent about it. Let's live from the heart; realize our heart is God, our heart is Buddha, our heart is capable of love and of effective achievement of whatever we set it on; and accept nothing less. And have a great time in the process!

Ruby Wax

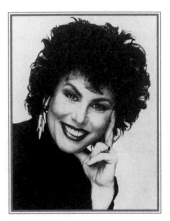

A writer, actress, and comedienne, Ruby Wax is famous for her outrageous documentaries and television interviews. Here she talks about her personal challenges and development and, in particular, her need for silence as she states, "In the silence I find my life worth living; I find it interesting. The rest of it is noise."

Free Falling

In comedy you can't break certain rules—it's a real technical thing—you need to deliver a punch line every so often. If there are too many gaps in a funny line, you lose your edge. That makes it difficult to stick to reality or to let any kind of message come through without always being a slave to the comedy. So I try to make my work about things that are a little wider; I try to have an underbelly in my comedy, to have a different issue underneath it. You have to do it really covertly if you've got a message, so it is difficult to combine being funny with your personal message.

I had a tricky home life, as many comedians do, so rather than go and complain about it, when no one would listen, I'd turn it into comedy. That way I could get attention and sympathy. Not being a particularly attractive girl, I got it any way I could! I thought I would be a great actress but there was no indication I could act. A big clue I couldn't act would have been that in my high school there were 6,000 chorus members of *Hello, Dolly!* and I didn't get a part! But I was like a bulldozer. I was rejected by every drama school except the Royal Scottish Academy in Glasgow, which wanted something a little rougher. It saw me and took me before I even finished my first sentence because I was a wild card. As soon as I got out, I said, "I'm going to the Royal Shakespeare Company," and I did.

I stayed for seven years, but I wasn't very good. Alan Rickman said, "You're very funny; write down what you think." So I started writing my own shows and putting all the stars of the company into the shows. I would play the lead, and Zoe Wannamaker would play; Alan Rickman or David Suchet would direct. And those shows were really funny. I never knew in all of high school and Berkeley University, where I got a C average in writing, that I could write, because they wouldn't let me free-fall. Alan made me free-fall in a way that my education had denied me.

My deeper stuff only started a few years ago. I'm really a late developer. Sex was late for me; everything was late. This is good because it means I age really slowly. Maybe it is good that I wasn't a great-looking girl; I wasn't even talented, and yet I decided I wanted to be an actress. There is a certain craziness to my life as well as denial. And sometimes denial is good; it means you jump off cliffs and have no fear.

I was doing those documentaries which are kind of free falling, called *Ruby Takes a Trip*. I wanted to go from the ridiculous to the profound, so I started off at the market end of the New Age in Los Angeles and spent three weeks talking to lunatics of every description. The most insane thing of all was when I married myself on the beach. Then I wanted to get as heavy as I could, so I met a guy who works with terminally ill kids and Vietnam vets and Native Americans. I did a vision quest with him. The first few days were in a sweat lodge where we did different rituals. I told the man leading us, Tom, that I thought we needed to stay critical so we could protect ourselves, but Tom remained steadfast without passing judgment.

Then I went off on my own in the woods for three days. The whole experience was kind of intense, but I went by myself—the cameras didn't follow me into the woods. Within a day I had changed from being scared of the dark to feeling as though the forest was watching over me, like a mother. There was this bigger presence over me, and I was more humbled than ever before in my life. Everything went very, very still and quiet within. As it got quieter, I began to see I had the potential to be much more interesting than I would be in the direction in which my mouth was leading me. Then, suddenly, I was aware of an aspect of God I had never before believed in: everywhere I looked the mundane became profound. I became a part of something very strong. I remember being able to concentrate on smaller and smaller objects and being able to stay with them.

Before we left, we had a final ritual in which we had to give away something important to us. I gave away my mirror, representing my vanity and my image on television. Then we had to say something about the journey, and I said that, for me, God was definitely in the details. And I talked about the parent in nature who was bigger than I.

At home I have a float tank, and when I've lost myself, I get in my tank. What's good about it is that even if you can't sit with yourself, you can always float. It's not about the tank and it's not about the water; it's about the silence. I need silence. Even when I was in the Royal Shakespeare Company, I would check into a hotel by myself for about three days and go into a kind of reverie without waking up, because too much fuel goes out of me too quickly. So I wouldn't call it anything spiritual, and people would laugh that I always had to be in a five-star hotel in order to meditate. Just because I'm on a spiritual journey doesn't mean I have to give up on room service! I like meditating, but I don't meditate on a word or anything specific. In the silence I find my life worth living; I find it interesting. The rest of it is noise. When we are silent something profound happens to individuals. I think that creating spaces for meditation is the only way that there is going to be any shift in the way we are, because we have all talked enough. Through the stillness something miraculous happens.

I really go for the high jolts of my job. I guess it's the bungee-jumping effect when you just jump off cliffs with no parachute. But if I didn't have a balance to that, I would go nuts. Then again if I lived in a small shack or hut all year round, I'd go nuts too. So it's somewhere between those two. One is right out there in front of the camera, and the other is in the silence.

I don't have a vision of the world, and I think I'm over my guilt that I don't. I think your own personal entanglement of wires that makes you work is so complex that it's enough that people should concentrate on themselves and then maybe send out a good ripple to the next person. Words like charity really fascinate me, because so many people do it for the wrong reasons. I always do AIDS, I'll always do cancer, I'll always do children's charity things. But I really cut a lot out because I have to ask why I am doing this; is it so I can show up at parties? I have to stop because there's a moment when I don't trust myself anymore. I have to tune in and say, "Does my heart connect to this one?"

Your whole life is trying to find a path, to figure out exactly when you're a lie to yourself. To me that's the only theme in my life—when am I a lie to myself? I find only a few people who work in a compassionate way, and me probably least of all. We're all really scared and trying to make ourselves more important than we are. I mean, nobody's putting down the mask and saying, "We're all crazy here aren't we?"

We've got some great thinkers, like the Dalai Lama. We've got these great guys out there, but for every one Mother Teresa we've got ten million schmucks. Is this the way whoever's in charge planned it? I think the news should be avoided because I don't even trust that anymore. You think just because you know someone was strangled in the forest, it is going to make you more compassionate? If everybody had a little bit of a mirror implant and saw themselves as they really are and if they were really honest about it, then that's when the healing would begin.

The world is not a mess here in this house, but it is two blocks away in the crack neighborhood. All you can do is look in yourself. I know when I go into my syndrome and I see the fear it creates. When I'm in my body and I'm centered, I see people full of love. I see the effect, that as I get more loving other people are softening around me, and that's about all I can do.

Satish Kumar

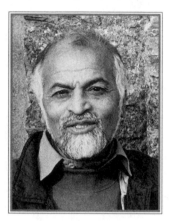

From being a Jain monk to walking from India to America, Satish Kumar has dedicated his life to peace through education by establishing the Small School and the Schumacher College, in Devon, England. The college, based on ecological and spiritual values, brings together teachers and students from around the globe. It is therefore no coincidence that he writes of the vital importance of community education. "Relationship is the basis of education. The book is not the basis; it is a tool."

The Heart of Education

From the age of nine I was a formal Jain monk in Rajistan. I left the monkhood at eighteen but informally I am still a Jain monk; this means that instead of practicing a formal Jain way of life, shut away from the world, I try to live the Jain way in everyday life. I learned from the Jain tradition compassion, truth, love, and nonviolence, and that always stays with me. But I was much inspired during my last years of monkhood by Gandhi, who said that it is no good dividing the world into monks and laypeople. When you are in a formal religious order, you easily get a feeling of holier-than-thouness; I'm a monk, I'm superior, and others are lower as they are laypeople and cannot reach the same heights of spirituality as a monk. Gandhi said that what we need is to bring truth, nonviolence, passion, consciousness, and spirituality into everyday life. In this way our politics would be informed by a spiritual ethos and value; our agriculture, business, industry, education, cooking, marriage—everything would be imbibed and informed by a deep spiritual source. "Ordinary" comes from the word *order,* so when you have perfect harmony and order in your life, then you are ordinary. I thought, this is a great challenge. How can you live an ordinary, informal life and practice spirituality?

I joined a Gandhian ashram after leaving the monkhood. I learned that when you are gardening, you look at the soil as sacred, and the plants growing out of that soil, and the seeds becoming plants—all have a sacred mystery and magic. You see the Divine in the soil, plants, trees, rivers, animals, people; everything is sacred. My mother embodied such awareness. She was a very wise yet simple person. She never studied in a school; she could not read, write, or sign her name. But she was a maker of beautiful things. Every morning when she awoke at four o'clock, before dawn, she would churn the butter while chanting and creating beautiful sounds of music. She would also make lovely embroidery with colorful threads. She would make a shawl with beautiful mirrorwork on it; then she would give this shawl away as a present. I remember my sister saying, "Mother, this shawl is so beautiful I cannot put it on my body; it will get dirty. I would like to put it on the wall as a hanging." Mother said, "When you start to put beautiful things on the wall you start to put ugly things on your body. Everything should be both beautiful and useful at the same time."

In 1962, when I was twenty-six years old, I took a journey walking for peace from India to Europe without any money. This took two and a half years. When you have money, you can be cut off from people; you can buy whatever you need—you can eat in a restaurant, you can sleep in a hotel, and you can move on the next day. When you have no money, you are totally vulnerable in the hands of those you meet; you have to depend on their generosity, kindness, and hospitality, and you have to take it as it comes. A true beggar, without money, has to accept what is given. So when you come to a town or a village, you look for people who are going to accept you and communicate with you and give you hospitality. Once you have that kind of relationship, you come in much closer contact with people, their families, their way of life, their ideas and culture, their religion. I needed very little transport on my walk, but people did raise funds to help me. Bertrand Russell helped me get to the United States from England, and Martin Luther King, Jr., helped me get from the United States to Japan, and so on.

Walking through Pakistan, Afghanistan, Iran, Armenia, Russia, Poland, Germany, France, England, the United States, and Japan and back to India, I found that whatever you are, you are primarily a human being. If you go as a Hindu, then you meet a Muslim. If you go as an Indian, then you meet a Pakistani or a Russian or an American; if you go as a Jain, then you meet a Christian. Divisions are our perception. So if you go as a humble human being, you meet human beings everywhere and there are no divisions.

Such a walk teaches you that trust is essential for relationship, for where there is no trust, there is no peace. I was proving that you can go into any culture, any country, and you can find humanity. So what is this problem of "I am a Catholic and you are a Protestant," "I am an Arab and you are a Jew," "I am Hindi, you are Muslim"? My name is Satish but I am not Satish. I am just a human being.

Some years later I was asked to come back to England to teach about nonviolence and to edit *Resurgence* magazine. Then, when my own son was about ten years old, I become deeply concerned and involved with education. We had come to live in a rural village, and I was confronted with having to send my son to a large school that was an hour's journey away. He would have become a commuter. The question that arose for me was, how can we have a community school that involves the whole village and the surrounding nature? I never went to a formal school, but I felt that the system was narrowing down the definition and concept of education to something called schooling, whereas I believed that education should be a living process that is happening all the time, that we are learning by being aware of all aspects of life, including nature, animals, plants, and divinity.

A number of people in the village agreed with me. They were

concerned that the kind of education their children would receive in the large school would be very reductionist, mechanistic, too formal and academic. In such schools you do not learn to use your hands, your heart, or your spirit; they are focused on intellectual information. We had a meeting and found we had nine children—enough to start a school. We bought a Methodist chapel in the village and started the Small School in 1982. We now have thirty children and over one hundred and fifty have graduated. The main principle is that the children should learn to create a community, that the school is like a learning community.

Now what is in the center of any community or house? It is the kitchen. So we said that in the Small School the kitchen would be the center of the school where the children and teachers would prepare the meals together. It is in the food we eat, in its nutritional value, in learning how to cook or how to serve it that we find our spirituality. In the Christian tradition, communion is sharing the bread together; the basis of communion is not some empty rhetoric but is bread and wine. We created a vegetable garden so the children could grow their own food. Education is spirituality, sharing, and community; they all come together. Around the growing and cooking of food, we have created a school in which the children learn mathematics, English, geography, and so on. These are added to the central core of the practical and spiritual aspects of education. I would like to see every school based on this central idea of school as community, in which students learn to share and to relate.

Relationship is the basis of education. The book is not the basis; it is a tool. The principle is relationship, with yourself, with who you are, with your fellow pupils, the teachers, your parents, and the community around you, and to the school building, the material, even the paper and pens—how you relate to these and respect them. Education shows you how to read but not what to read. I believe education should show you how to read; it should tell you what to read, and also tell you why to read. Reading is not the source of all knowledge; we need to learn through all our senses—touching, tasting, smelling, hearing, seeing—by being with people, and by respecting our world.

Our children pass exams with flying colors, with few problems. We see the exams as only a small matter, with none of the anguish and stress that affects other schools and their students. They make so much of exams, whereas the entry into life and society is a bigger matter. Because we are stimulating our children at the Small School in this more complete way, they are passing their exams with no trauma, no problem. Exams are not seen as a horror or a nightmare. We say to the children, "Don't worry; you will pass. What is most important is to learn about life."

When there is no fear, then it is natural to be competent on exams. Children are normally so frightened, and where fear rules, education cannot take place. Education cannot be based on fear of exams, teachers, parents, school, or being bullied or punished. Education should be ruled by trust and love and respect. This is a totally different philosophy.

There should be a Small School in every community, every neighborhood. No school should have more than one or two hundred children. When children don't know their community, their teachers, their fellow pupils, the school becomes like a factory in which the children become like numbers and from which they all come out the same with no individuality or skills. Children should be able to interact with their teachers with confidence and trust.

As a society we have such a narrow view of education; we develop the intellectual so that the student can get a job and compete. I want us to see the bigger picture that includes the whole person. Economics is important, but there is more to life than economic growth. Our government, business, and industry are so focused on economic growth that they exclude the spiritual and artistic and imaginative growth. There is so little time given to developing hand skills—how to make things, how to mend things, how to grow things, how to cook, how to build. There is so much head and so little heart. I want to see a child's education developing all the senses and, beyond them, the spirit.

When I started the Small School many people asked about adult education as, certainly, education does not stop at the end of our formal schooling. So I proposed the idea for a college to the Dartington Trust, and with their support we formed the Schumacher College. People come for three to five weeks to live together, to cook and clean and learn together. There are no servants, no staff to do the chores, because there is no way we can say that I am learning great spiritual ideals while someone else is cleaning my toilet; it has to be holistic. All the participants and staff cook, clean, meditate, learn, study, garden, go on field trips—everything connected and together.

There are many creative and radical thinkers in the environmental, ecological, scientific, literary, and humanistic fields who are deeply spiritual and holistic in their understanding, but their work is not recognized by mainstream academia. So we provide a place where they can come to live with their family and with the participants for a few weeks at a time. And it works wonderfully.

Indian philosophy is based on the belief that the Divine and creation are not different; the dancer and the dance cannot be separated. There is no dualism. For me, nature, humans, and the Divine are totally interlinked, entwined. I want to make Schumacher College an educational center in which humans, nature, and the Divine can be united together. That is the challenge. Without nature, you cannot have social cohesion; without social cohesion, you cannot care for nature. Without social cohesion and nature, there is no Divine, and without divinity and spirituality, society will go bankrupt. So you cannot separate this trinity; education is to see the unity.

My intent is that we should see that education is not confined to the four walls of the schools and colleges. We should liberate it from the formalities of formal education, from being a tool for economic or industrial purposes, so it can be for the full growth and development and unfoldment of human potential and spirit. The big picture is to see each human being making a full contribution to the development of society, which includes spiritual, artistic, and environmental development, as well as economic. We need to eat and work, but economics should not be given importance to the exclusion of other development. Then education can fulfill its whole meaning. Education is essential; we learn all the time and we are never too old. We are simply learning to be who we really are.

Peter Goldfarb

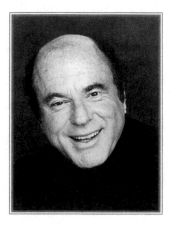

A philanthropist, actor, director, and producer who is deeply involved with the spiritual journey, Peter Goldfarb delights in bringing greater authenticity to acting through discovering the manifold aspects of the self. Here he shares how that authenticity brings transformation. "By facilitating each individual to access his or her own extraordinary uniqueness," he says, "there can be a transcendence of the habitual through the function of authenticity."

Passionate Creativity

I first began as a performer when I was quite young; when I was just eighteen I started directing and at twenty-two I produced my first play. When it came time to make a decision about my career, I looked at what the life of an actor was like and I wasn't inspired. I saw what I would call "poverty mentality": everything from literal poverty, in which actors have to scrape and struggle from one job to another to survive, to the psychological realm of poverty, in which actors feel an external dependence for a sense of fulfillment or satisfaction. I also saw a lot of ego—a quality of being both inflated and defensive at the same time. I saw this in myself, yet I also felt very insecure, and that insecurity was part of the vulnerability that nurtured me as an actor. If I thought I was wonderful, where was I going to go or how could I grow?

The ostensible dependency of an actor comes from the fact that you have to audition and somebody has to like you so you get hired, or you are not liked and are refused the part; who you are or how you are is not acceptable. It seems so much of our culture is conditioned by the programming of our being incomplete, as if something is absent inside and therefore we have to focus on getting it from outside. Like the commercials that carry the message that you need a certain deodorant, car, or designer label, so the actor needs someone to approve, accept, or acknowledge him or her. Everywhere I looked I saw this programmed dependency. If the assumption is that that's just the way it has to be, how can it be possible not to be dependent?

Later I began to understand that performance, for me, had nothing to do with either building myself up or feeling dependent. It had to do with manifesting a sense of generosity: if this is my gift, if this is what I am most capable of doing, then it is also the way I can most touch other people's lives. Within that context I experience myself as a kind of vehicle through which something flows and manifests. Something happens when we follow our passion, and the result is this expression of generosity; if people receive it that way, it is a gift that touches their lives. It isn't about constructing and solidifying ego; it's about manifesting compassion and generosity.

The answer to dependency, I believe, lies in shifting from the conditioned allegiance to dependency, to a conscious allegiance to the process of self-empowerment. Through my experience with many varied disciplines not directly related to acting, I began to synthesize a process of creative empowerment which, at the very least, redressed the imbalance between external dependency and self-realization or creative fulfillment. For instance, an actor thinks she or he has to go to school to learn how to speak or move properly, how to learn technique, and so on. In almost all our educational systems there is this hidden dependency: I can't be a good actor unless I learn how to do this or that. But what about each individual's organic sense of movement and speech, our authentic way of being in the world? Normally we learn through imitating what we see and hear; we are not necessarily walking or talking the way our own bodies were meant to. Yet we are organisms, each differentiated in a unique fashion.

By facilitating each individual to access his or her own personal and very extraordinary uniqueness, there can be a transcendence of the habitual through the fruition of authenticity. When the individual begins to have an experience of her authentic self and of the creative resources at her disposal, that in itself is transformation. As such, I don't see performance as a need to be seen; I experience it more in terms of my willingness to allow my being to be seen. This means that I open in such a way that what is supposed to come through me will come through. The process of preparing a role to me is one of gradually but insistently removing myself as an obstacle. If I go into a situation believing that I know something, then this inhibits my spontaneity; I have a prior reference point and I am not there in the moment with the situation as it is. So I am both committed to the search and to not knowing.

Rather than define the creative process, I prefer to respond to its continual challenge to remain open and fresh. One such challenge I set for myself as a teacher was to see how far I could go without teaching any technique whatsoever. The amazing thing is that, appropriately nurtured and facilitated, each actor's speech or movement emerges fully formed. So it isn't even a question of bad or good. It's like Venus coming out of the water, Athena being born from the head of Zeus, fully formed. If a performer is coming from something that he himself has engendered, then it is a given that his commitment is total because he is not struggling to imitate any kind of model outside of himself.

I work with guided fantasy and dreams, experiential exercises that bypass the cerebral and the conceptual mind. There is an exercise I do that begins as a guided fantasy, in which you imagine yourself as a member of the opposite sex. You imagine how your body feels, what you are wearing, what your occupation is, and what you are doing. You ask if you have hobbies, if you have a boyfriend or girlfriend. You become the person. This isn't difficult because you already know everything you need to know about this person; you have created the person directly from a place where you haven't had to think—the creative unconscious. It is remarkable to see the characters that people come up with and to witness how we all walk around with these characters inside ourselves.

I believe that becoming oneself is the true transcendence, because what one is transcending is the limited view of oneself, the self that is defined by ego. This is not the same as throwing out the ego. The problem with ego is when we think that's all there is and identify only with it; we buy into the result and start to believe our own image. That is what causes so much suffering and confusion with success, whether as an actor or as something else, such as a spiritual teacher. There is a difference between how we are and how people respond to how we are, particularly if the response is conditioned by dependency. If I resonate with someone and say, "Yes, this is an appropriate model for me," that helps me in my own process. But if I say, "This person is going to save me," I am perpetuating that dependency. Then I will begin to project qualities of authority or enlightenment onto that person. And sometimes, depending on who he or she is, that person will believe all this attention and buy into the image of savior.

Everybody has a practice; some people practice meditation, some practice neurosis. If we are suffering, then our practice is suffering; if we come to a point where we understand we are not our suffering, then we cease to practice suffering and move onto a more self-nurturing practice. I am not attributing something either wonderful or not wonderful to practice. Why would I be great by practicing meditation and not be great by practicing piano playing? But we tend to associate practice with something spiritual and special. I think that the sooner we understand that everyone is practicing something, the easier it is to move toward the kind of awareness that leads to more self-empowerment, to compassionate and generous practice.

I've had the opportunity to observe and experience the enormous richness of the human spirit, to watch people transform as they begin to understand that all they need to do is to be who they are, be their authentic human self. The word spiritual seems to engender duality because it implies there must be nonspiritual. To me being is about understanding that we do not have to worry about getting this and that or learning this and that, because there is no this and that; it's just about getting in touch with our own inimitable and infinite creative resources.

There is a tendency to resist the understanding and awareness of our authenticity because it seems so simple, but the creative experience is there in every moment. It's simply a matter of shifting our allegiance, our identification, to see that there is very little we need to do and that judgments or comparisons are futile. The differences or distinctions are only those of form. There is the form of the theater, of the play, of the character, and of the act, in the same way as there are all the different forms of our life. We change according to the form: if a bomb were to drop into my living room right now, my behavior would change. I would respond to that form. However, these are only forms, and we don't have to confuse the form with the process, the content with the essence. There are forms within which it is possible for us to manifest more fully than within other forms. I can express myself more fully as a performer than I could driving a bus, but for some people it's the opposite. There are some wonderful characters driving buses because they have found the form in which they can most manifest themselves.

We need to bury the illusion that we even have a choice of being anything other than what we are. Rather than all this confusion of what should I do with my life, I feel we need to ask, what am I truly passionate about, where is my passion? When we respond to our passion then we can never be anything other than who we are.

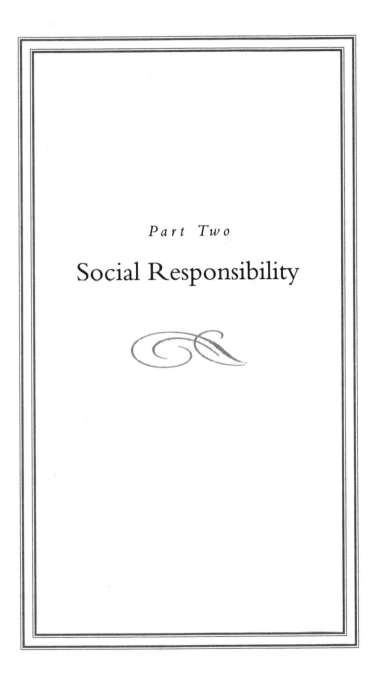

Part Two

Social Responsibility

Rama Vernon

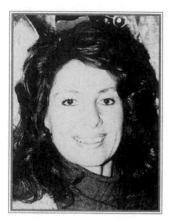

*W*hile *the editor of the* Yoga Journal, *Rama Vernon found herself catapulted into the world of Russian-American politics. As a result of her subsequent efforts, thousands have partici-pated in Soviet-American Citizens Sum-mits through the Center for International Dialogue, founded by Rama. Here she shares her story and, in particular, the words of wisdom she received from a Rus-sian colleague: "Bravery does not mean you are without fear. It means you have the courage to face your fear."*

A Leap of Faith

In 1984 I was invited by the late Danaan Parry of the Earth Stewards group to travel with thirty others on a peace mission to the Soviet Union. The Cold War was at its peak. The Korean Airlines disaster had recently occurred, bringing us very close to a nuclear war. All sports, educational, and arts exchanges were cut off between our countries, and we lived with a growing dread of an impending clash with the other superpower. As I put my children to bed at night, they would ask, "Mommy, are we going to be blown up?" "No, of course not," I would reply, reassuring them as much as myself. "Our government would never let that happen."

I accepted the invitation to the U.S.S.R. and, in preparation, attended a luncheon held by a highly respectable Seattle organization. They were hosting three Soviets who represented the Institute for Canadian-American Studies in Moscow: Dr. Henry Trofimenko, head of foreign relations for the U.S.S.R.; Alla Bobrysheva, vice president of the institute; and Dr. Luv Karpov, a leading Soviet economist. The institute, equivalent to the CIA, was known for its training of Soviet intelligence agents, so I was excited. They would be the first Russians I had ever met; it would be a preliminary glimpse behind the Iron Curtain. Also being hosted was Dr. Abraham Ysrael of the U.S. State Department. "How wonderful," I erroneously thought. "They will be able to dialogue." Even though I knew nothing about politics, it didn't take a Sovietologist to realize that dialogue was not on the agenda, at least not on the part of the United States.

During the meeting, Dr. Trofimenko would start to speak and our State Department representative would continually interrupt in a rather bombastic and argumentative way. This tactic obstructed any possibility of dialogue and was an embarrassment to the Soviet guests and the hosting organization, as well as to members of the audience. This was not dialogue. It was open confrontation. It felt as if I were awakening from a slumber into the realization that our government, which I had always thought had its people's best interest at heart, did not want to end the Cold War. Until then, I had thought the Soviet Union was responsible for its own political isolation; now I saw a different picture. A chill ran through my body. It was a startling realization for one who had always trusted. I couldn't sit there any longer, so I excused myself and went to the ladies' room. Perhaps, I thought hopefully, this is just overreaction on my part. Since I know nothing of politics, maybe there is something I am missing here.

The attempts to reassure myself were short-lived. The ladies' room was filled with politically astute women venting their own fears after witnessing this aborted dialogue. Eyes were wide with confusion and concern for our future. That day at the luncheon I made a commitment to myself. "I am a U.S. citizen and I am as responsible for the peace between the United States and the U.S.S.R. as the officials of my government. There has to be something an ordinary citizen can do to avert our Cold War stereotypes from escalating," I thought, while wondering how a wife and mother could do anything. It seemed impossible, but I knew I had to try.

Two months later I left for the U.S.S.R. On the first day in Moscow our group visited the Soviet Peace Committee. We were brought into a hugely imposing room with large, glossy tables that had translation microphone equipment at every seat. The representatives were impressively lined up at the head tables. I was conditioned to believe, like every American, that they were the enemy—the Communist devils—and that we were not to believe anything they said. It was surprising to later learn that only 6 to 10 percent of the Soviet population were card-carrying Communists and even those were quick to whisper (unofficially) their anger and disillusionment with the system.

The Soviet Peace Committee representatives looked like ducks standing in a row. The men wore leather jackets while the women reinforced our post-World War matronly stereotype. My skepticism flowered. "I bet they are all KGB agents and this is a front for the government." It was only many years later that I found out I was right.

I remember that first day at the Peace Committee so clearly. The representatives spoke about their work and then asked if there were any questions. Members from our group would ask, "What about your policy in Afghanistan?" and they would ask back, "What about your policy in Vietnam?" Another of our group would ask, "What about your human rights?" and they would say, "What about your civil rights?"

Wait a minute, I thought, this is not dialogue. This is what happened at the meeting in Seattle; this doesn't work. There has to be another way; we have to somehow do this differently. I sat there asking for guidance. What could I do to help end the Cold War? And the thought came: bring a thousand people to come and see these people as people; arrange a meeting where there is a one-on-one dialogue that is based on collaboration, harmony, and cooperation, not on arguments, judgments, and debate.

The next day I was in Red Square and had another revelation. Seeing all the guards marching like Hitler's armies, and the red star on the Kremlin, I started to quiver with fear, because I saw how I had been conditioned to believe that these people were the enemy. I was standing in the center of what Reagan had termed the Evil Empire and behind what Churchill had called the Iron Curtain. I was in the heart of the territory of the enemy. But I was also raised to believe that our thoughts create our reality, so I realized that what scared me most was that I was not alone in my fear of the Evil Empire, that hundreds of thousands of Americans shared those same fears with me and that if enough of us continued to hold those fears, we would create the thing that we feared most. We would create these people as our enemy.

So that day I thought, "How can I change this?" The only way to change a stereotype that we have been conditioned to believe is to bring people face to face with one another. We couldn't take the Russians to the United States; they were not allowed to travel unless they were screened by the KGB. So I thought, "If they can't travel, we will travel. I'll bring thousands of Americans here to look into their faces."

I realized that first I should meet the Russian people myself. So on that first trip, through all the different republics we visited, I made an effort to connect with each person I met. I had the most miraculous experience of looking into the eyes of these people I had been taught to believe were the enemy, and I saw only the friend. I had one very distinct experience in Georgia, in Tblisi, in the marketplace early one morning. A woman came up to me and said "Italiana?" I said, "No, American." She cried out, "American! American!" Groups of people started gathering around. She dropped to her knees, her hands in prayer position, and with tears in her eyes started pleading and begging me for peace. "Mir . . . Mir . . ." I helped her stand up and we just held each other and cried.

When I returned to the United States from that first trip it was a turning point. I made a proposal that a hundred Americans come and meet with a hundred Soviet counterparts, in the fields of education, health, economics, and the environment. American Airlines said it would donate tickets. In Connecticut I met the representative of the Soviet Peace Committee to give him the proposal. I had no idea what I was doing; all I knew was that I had to do something for my children and all future generations. I did not trust that our government would make the right decisions in those moments that would stop the Cold War. I felt that if we, the people, wanted to make a change, we each had to be responsible.

When I met the Soviet official, my hand was trembling because I thought he was going to say this proposal was the most ridiculous thing that he had ever seen. But he looked at it and tears came into his eyes, and when he put it down, he said, "This is just what the doctor ordered." He loved the idea of the one-on-one contact. He said, "We can play volleyball together!" And then I understood that they had as much of a hunger to come together with us as we had to come together with them.

It was a very long journey from there to organizing the first trip. It took a year, and then after that we were doing sometimes six or seven trips a year, and pretty soon every month. I felt we needed to bring people en masse—the largest group we took was two hundred and fifty people—and to bring people of heart, those with a deep spiritual understanding, who also had academic credentials because the Soviet authorities really respect credentials. And I felt that we should dress with respect and not wear sandals or Levi's, as I knew they would then take us more seriously. The Sufis have a saying, "The more far out you are, the straighter your cover should be." So I bought my first pair of nylons in years; I bought the wardrobe and really started to gain respect and entrance into the labyrinth of the Soviet system. And it was a labyrinth. But I got through doors in a way that I was told later seemed like the parting of the Red Sea!

I was having to commute over there because there was no reliable phone connection. You had to book a call three days ahead; there was no central switchboard. There was no Federal Express, no computers. But slowly we broke into more and more avenues and higher echelons of the Soviet system. I knew that those held the people we had to reach. I didn't even know that there was a law at that time against foreigners going into Russian homes or that the Soviets could not have contact with foreigners; I just knew instinctively that we had to have U.S. people connect with as many Russian people as they could so that they would know we were not the enemy. It was very profound. We touched hundreds of thousands of lives.

On my twenty-fourth visit, one of the Soviet leaders said, "Your next visit is your silver anniversary; we must arrange something very special for you." The next time I came back I was bringing the Global Family Group for their first trip. President Ronald and Nancy Reagan were in Moscow for the second summit with President Mikhail Gorbachev, and I was invited to a tea that was being hosted by Raisa Gorbachev for Nancy Reagan. And then, the next day, I and two of my colleagues were invited to be part of a special meeting in the Kremlin with President Gorbachev. I had a gift for President Gorbachev, a ten-ton monument of two hands coming together from the marble quarries of Italy. This signified the ratification of the peace treaty between our two countries at that time.

When it was my turn to speak, I said, "I have a picture here to present to you, but I cannot present the gift in person because it is fifteen feet high and weighs ten tons." The whole room burst into laughter, and President Gorbachev said, "Do you think it is too big for us to handle?" When I gave him the picture, he took my hand, and I felt like I had been working from the bottom up while he had been working from the top down and at that moment our hands touched. That day I rededicated myself to peace. I had given myself one year to work for peace, and by this time four years had gone by. That day I dedicated my whole life to working toward peaceful solutions.

The reason why I was brought to that meeting was because we put on the first Soviet-American Citizens Summit in Washington, D.C. , from the end of 1987 to February 1988. We hosted a hundred top-level Soviets in Washington, D.C., and put on a conference with them and with five hundred Americans called the First Soviet-American Citizens Summit: Social Inventions for the Third Millennium. By this time I had realized that it wasn't enough just to take Americans to Russia. Certainly they had heartfelt openings and loved the Russians. They came back and spoke at churches and Rotary Clubs and this helped to change people's stereotypes. But when we put on the Citizens Summit, it was a major turning point in Soviet-American relations.

Russians are very deeply spiritual people but they had been totally repressed. We were the first ones who started bringing officials into the church, testing the limits. We brought in Ukrainian Russian Bibles and opened them up to Customs which read them and then let us go through. It was really miraculous what was transpiring. The Russian people were hungry because their spirituality had gone underground.

We ended up with two offices, one in Kiev and one in Moscow. When the war between Armenia and Azerbaijan started, Max (my partner) and I were asked by the Soviet government to go in and create some kind of resolution between the two countries. It was very hard, but people who would not even look at each other to begin with, after the first day were like brothers coming together.

We closed our office in the Soviet Union in 1991 because the Cold War was over and we felt that our work was done. On the last visit in 1990 one of Gorbachev's people said, "You have laid down your life, everything, for our people. You love our people so much you have given us everything. People have tried to stop you and pull the rug from under you, or stab you in the back just like they did with Gorbachev, but you kept going and didn't let anything stop you. And now our people are free. The people that you have brought here are the best of America, the heart of America. You have brought the people of heart that have opened our hearts." Yet at the same time there was a great depression there. People were flocking to the cities in search of food. There was no heating in our big office. We were sitting in our gloves and coats and we could see our breath in the air, and I was afraid even to cry because I thought my tears might freeze. I said, "I feel sad because the people are hungry." But he said, "Your mission here was to free our people, not to feed our people."

In 1990 we, as the Center for International Dialogue, were asked to go to Israel to work with the Israelis and Palestinians, and we were asked to work with the Ethiopians. The need for dialogue between people is urgent, to come together across the boundaries that we set for ourselves and the boundaries that our governments set, to expand the parameters of the mind, to come together to learn to trust, to overcome our fear of one another by looking into each other's eyes. How can we hold fear of that with which we are familiar?

I didn't plan to help the world. I was raised in the Eastern disciplines of Yoga and meditation, feeling that it was every man for himself. You liberate yourself; you come to the place where you see the world as an illusion. I've seen the particles that make up these atoms we call solid. And I'd always thought that if I could just meditate and find my own peace, that was the greatest gift that I could give to the world. When the whole Russian thing started, I really agonized over it, especially when they accepted the first proposal. I knew that my whole life would change. I knew that it meant leaving my family, leaving everything that was dear to me and familiar, that it was the pilgrim's path. I was stepping out like a warrior, stepping to the edge.

No one spoke about the edge in those days, but I kept having this vision that I was going through these jungle paths, cutting away at the underbrush, and all of a sudden I came to the edge of a cliff. When I looked out, the other side was far away, and when I looked back, the path behind me had closed. I was standing on the edge with a chasm of darkness below, and the other side was so far away that it would take a quantum leap of consciousness to reach it. Sometimes my head would hurt; I felt my skull couldn't move fast enough for my brain to expand. I just felt I had to take this giant leap. And I knew I had to lighten my burden before I made that leap. I had this vision for four months over and over, that I was on the edge of the cliff and the vision was requiring me to leap over the chasm of consciousness of the unknown.

I remember the day when I finally gathered all my strength and morale, everything I had in me after years of discipline—yogic discipline, advanced practice, meditation, breathing—and even then I didn't know if I had the courage. I gathered it all up, and I remember taking this leap knowing I couldn't possibly stretch far enough to reach the other side. But I had to. So I jumped, and I didn't fall. An invisible hand was there to hold me. It held me tenderly as it carried me across the chasm. I don't know how I got to this other place of consciousness, but I crossed an enormous boundary of fear inside myself.

You don't do this work unless you're going to give everything. In later years the Soviet generals whom I dealt with called me the "brave woman" because I went there four times while I was pregnant, then I brought my three-month-old daughter. I was nursing my baby, writing notes with one hand and holding her with the other. Every door seemed to open to me because the mother has a great significance in the old orthodox beliefs. They put us on television because they couldn't get over this U.S. woman traveling with a newborn baby across the oceans to come to them.

They kept saying, "You're such a brave woman." One day I said to one of my Soviet colleagues, "I'm not brave. When I started this work, my knees would tremble with fear. Not of you all, but of the fear of making a mistake that might hurt the people." He said,

"Bravery does not mean you are without fear. It means you have the courage to face your fear."

Going on the front lines became my spiritual practice. What we do in Yoga is take a posture and become familiar with it, and then we go to the next posture, which represents the unknown. Then that becomes the known, and we take another variation which is the unknown. So we're always expanding the parameters of our consciousness until there are no boundaries. But it was the most difficult practice I've had to do. My definition of faith is grace under pressure.

After the first Russian trip my marriage broke up. I came back from Russia on thin air, knowing I had no money to sustain this work. I had no idea how to continue. On the plane I moved my seat three times to get away from people smoking. Finally I was put up front and the only extra seat on the plane was next to me. As we started pulling away from the gate, I said a prayer. "Dear God, I feel I am to continue to do this work. But I have nothing left; there are no funds, no support, nothing. If you want me to do this work, you must provide a way for me to come back." That was my call.

As soon as I had finished, the plane stopped and went back to the gate; they opened the door and a man got on. There were no other seats available, so he sat down next to me. Since he was an American, I asked him what he was doing in Russia, as at that time very few Americans went there. And he said, "I'm the northwest representative for Finnair." By the end of that plane journey I had all the free tickets I needed to get back to Russia and to take groups, and Finnair even gave us our first computer and letterhead. It sponsored us for about a year. Each time we needed a new sponsor, one would come along. Pretty soon the work became self-sustainable, and we built in a small administrative fee for group trips that financially sustained us.

I feel all of us have a responsibility to expand our service, not just for our own inner salvation but into the world around us in whatever way we can. Never say no. When we say yes, we open new doors to new universes, to what our true service is to be. It may not always look like what we think we're supposed to be doing, but it will lead us to our life purpose. When I took that first step, I didn't know where it would lead; I didn't know that it would take me to other countries, that I would be involved as a peacemaker. If we really believe we are one, then we will know that the cry of that hungry child in Africa or that dying child in Russia is our child, and that those we bomb are our own. If our boundaries dissolve into seeing our world as a global family, we can never make war on another. Open your heart to feel the suffering of others as you feel your own. See others as yourself. And eventually you will see that there are no others.

At the U.N. World Women's Conference in Beijing we sat in a circle with women from Somalia, and we listened to their pain, we shared their grief, we held their hands. We dove into the sea of this suffering while we held the vision of a healed world, a healed country, a healed family. We held the vision of seeing them no longer as the walking dead, as they call these women who have lost their husbands, children, everything. They are alive in body but dead in their souls. After we sat with them, the women from Somalia and Rwanda said, "We feel so happy. We don't have any reason to feel happy, but we feel happy in our hearts." And I felt that if we could give them that gift in two minutes out of their lives, that's a great gift. For them to know they're supported and loved by sisters who really care, that gives such hope. They said, "You have given us hope, you have given us energy, you have given us strength to go back and make the changes we must make."

I used to believe that the world is an illusion so why do anything, but now I know that if we go on believing like that, then the karmic wheel just keeps turning. We not only have our individual karma, we have a national karma, we have a global karma. If we let human rights violations continue from one group to another, then we are perpetuating the problem in our inaction. But if we go into the situation in anger, we also perpetuate the problem. If we do our inner work and can stay in that center and then do the work that presents itself to us—whatever we are being called upon to do—whether it's in our home, community, or nation or in other countries in the world, then it moves toward a solution.

Millard Fuller

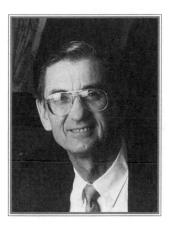

After he became a self-made millionaire, Millard Fuller gave away his money
and founded Habitat for Humanity International, a Christian housing ministry
that has provided affordable housing for
thousands of people worldwide. In this
piece he shares his personal journey and
the extraordinary work of Habitat: "You
can focus on the tremendous need and get
discouraged or you can focus on what is
going right, like building a house every
fifty minutes."

A House Every Fifty Minutes

I was in business with a fellow student at the University of Alabama. We worked together for three years in law school, and then after law school for five years in Montgomery. We worked day and night, literally, for eight years, to generate the huge amount of money that we made. But what I did in the process of this headlong rush to material success was go off and leave my wife. I didn't physically leave her, in the sense of separating from her; we had our home together. But I left her emotionally, and I left her in the evenings. I would come home, eat supper, and then go back to the office, and sometimes I would stay at the office all night, come home and eat breakfast, and then go back to work. The consequence was that we drew apart. She ended up leaving me, saying that she was considering a divorce, that we had no marriage, that the love relationship was over. I had ensconced her in a beautiful home with a maid; she had as much money as she could possibly want, a Lincoln Continental to drive around, a cabin on the lake, speedboats, horses—everything but a husband. It was that shocking event of her leaving me that caused me to reevaluate my life, because I loved her dearly.

I realized that I had gained all this material success, but I was about to lose the one thing that was so incredibly special to me.

Eventually we met in New York for a tearful reunion, with a lot of confession and honesty, and as we started back to the hotel, the idea came to me that we should simply give all our money away and start over. We were in a taxi cab, and as I shared this idea with Linda, I felt a sensation of light fill the cab. It was not some mysterious thing, just a sensation of light. I told Linda that I felt God was involved in our lives and that I felt we were being called to divest ourselves of our fortune, to give our money away and make ourselves poor again, so that we could draw closer to one another and closer to God. She never questioned that.

We went back to our hotel room and called up the pastor who had been counseling her. We told him that we had started the process of reconciliation and that one of the things we wanted to do was to give all our money away. He was shocked by that and counseled us not to do it. He told us that it was a rash decision made in the heat of emotion and that we should talk about it in the morning. We said no, that we knew it was illogical and that if we thought about it, we wouldn't do it. So we wanted to commit to him that that was what we were going to do.

The next morning when we left the hotel, we got into the first taxi that came by. Instead of just driving away, the taxi driver turned and said to us, "Congratulations. This is a brand new taxi; no one has ever ridden in it before." We saw that as confirmation from God that we had made the right decision, and we have never wavered in that decision nor regretted it in any way. We had chosen to start anew.

We don't advocate that this is what everybody else should do, but as practicing Christians, we know that it is very difficult for the rich to get into the Kingdom. We were very active in church, and previously, like most people, I had rationalized our money by saying, "Oh, sure, I've got a lot of money, but I'm willing to give it away. It's just that I don't feel God has called on me to give it away, so in the meantime I'm very rich and I live in a big house with servants and drive a big car. But if God ever told me to give it away, I would." I do believe now that we cannot serve both God and money, although I have known some wealthy people who have had a good balance in their lives, who were not controlled by their money. They had somehow been able to do a very difficult thing—to remain humble and dependent on God even though they had a lot of money.

The Bible says that with God all things are possible. So I've got to say that even a millionaire can be a Christian. But it is very difficult—not impossible but difficult. When you have a lot of money, why do you need to trust God? You trust your money; it will take care of everything. If you want to go on a trip, you buy a ticket. Money is the center of your life. That was the case for me, and my wife and I both felt that we needed to get rid of that which had separated us from each other and from God.

After a couple of years working with one of our church-related colleges, we moved to Koinonia Farm, a small Christian community near Americus, Georgia. During a month-long visit there right after we had left the business, we talked lots about faith, about Christianity, and about what is important, and I was just blown away by this guy Clarence Jordan, who was running the place. I had never seen anyone who was so committed or who had such keen insights into the Bible. We stayed in touch after we left, but during the next two years he said that the community looked like it might have to close; they had been shot at, dynamited, and jailed because they had African Americans and whites working and living together. He had told some of the African American people in the area that when they closed down Koinonia, they would sell them some lots so that they could at least have some land, and maybe one day they could get some money to build a house. We moved there to see if we could help keep the community going.

We started talking about how we could make our faith relevant, what we could do to be relevant Christians. We saw so many church people who seemed irrelevant. All they did was go to church and sit down and sing a few hymns and go home and live their lives as usual; they made no real contribution to the community. So we started talking about how we could make a difference, and we came up with the idea of partnership farming, partnership industries, and partnership housing. We started some small businesses for the community, and then we started building houses for the poor people in the area who had no other way to get a house.

While we still had the first house under construction, Clarence Jordan unexpectedly died. He was fifty-seven years old and I was thirty-one, and there I was with this dream. I stuck with it and stayed there nearly five years building houses for and with the poor. We were sufficiently excited by the success of this that I wanted to test it out in a developing country. So we went to Zaire (now the Democratic Republic of the Congo), where we had been a few years earlier, and built houses there for three years. And it was while I was in Africa that I realized that this little concept that we were dealing with, of getting people to help build houses and then selling them to the families at no profit and no interest, that this simple idea had worldwide implications. So I came back to the United States in 1976 with that dream in my heart, and being a lawyer, I incorporated a nonprofit charitable corporation called Habitat for Humanity and we invited the world to join us.

It is now over twenty-one years since that happened. We are in fifty-four countries and more than two thousand cities, towns, and villages; we build a house every fifty minutes and have built over sixty thousand so far. It's just an idea that took off and caught hold. All this started by building just one house for one needy family. Then we took it to Africa, and then we brought it back from Africa; and then I went to Guatemala and we got it started in Guatemala, and then to Uganda, and then to Peru. Meanwhile we kept going from city to city in the United States, spreading by word of mouth.

A Habitat for Humanity house in Haiti does not look at all like one in Atlanta, Georgia, or New York City. We build a simple, decent house within the context of where it is located. We are in over one thousand four hundred cities in the United States; we have built about twenty thousand houses here. Each city is responsible for raising the money. In third world countries we give a lot more help. The theory is that in countries like England or Canada, poverty is surrounded by wealth, but in a place like the Congo, poverty is surrounded by more poverty. Each local group has its own requirements, but the two main criteria that we use are that a person is living in inadequate housing and that he or she is too poor to get conventional financing.

We operate by what I call the "theology of the hammer." Two basic ideas underlie this theology. The first idea is that true religion has to be more than singing and talking. If you think about it, religion is normally expressed through listening to preaching, attending Sunday school class, praying, and chanting or singing. But the theology of the hammer says that there must be another dimension for it to be holistic and authentic and that that dimension must be an action component. So the theology of the hammer is the action component of religion. And within the context of Habitat it means you've got to take the hammer and hit the nail to make a house for somebody to live in, because one of the teachings of Jesus is to invite strangers in. He said that inasmuch as you do it to one of the least, you do it to me.

The second idea is that the theology of the hammer brings together a wide array of people. We are not Protestant, we are not Catholic, we are not liberal, we are not conservative. We've got African Americans and whites building houses together, we've got former guerrillas and government people building together in El Salvador, and we've got Protestants and Catholics building together in Northern Ireland. So Habitat is also a reconciling force. Where else would you see a former president of the United States (Jimmy Carter) building a house with a truck driver?

We turn hundreds, even thousands of unskilled volunteers loose on a work site, and somebody will tell them what to do. Habitat for Humanity is a not-for-profit organization, so the people working have no motivation for cutting corners. They typically build the houses extremely well because of pride in workmanship and a desire to make sure that the family who is going to live there is going to get a good house. Most times they put in twice the number of nails needed just to make sure the house is a good one!

There is a huge number of people in inadequate homes, and the job of getting them adequate housing is enormous. But you can focus on the tremendous need and get discouraged or you can focus on what is going right, like building a house every fifty minutes. I could psych myself up to be depressed and get discouraged if I just focused on the great need and on our seemingly small resources, but I take great strength in knowing that with God all things are possible. I believe that if we do a lot of little things right, they'll have a way of growing into big things.

Typically we build in poor neighborhoods, in places that are devastated. So when we build a Habitat house, everybody is delighted, because it is a nice house going up in a place where everybody has terrible houses. But in some of the more affluent cities in which we build, the neighbors typically have two big fears. Firstly, they fear that if we build these modest houses, it is going to make their house values go down. And, secondly, some people have the idea that all poor people are crooks, that if a person is poor, she or he is probably a prostitute, drug addict, alcoholic, or child molester. And they don't want such people living close to them. So they get very angry and say, "We don't want these people here. We don't know who they are, but they are bad people and we don't want them living next to us."

There are various ways you can deal with this. In Florida, when the neighbors rose up in righteous anger, the new home owners there went knocking door to door. When the neighbor came to the door, they would say, "I'm so-and-so. I'm going to be living in one of the houses here, and I'm the person you don't like. I want you to meet me. I'm not that bad." And they won them over.

When we got land for about thirty houses in a neighborhood in Washington, D.C., the neighbors all rose up in anger. Carol Casperson is a gutsy woman who runs our Washington, D.C., affiliate. Carol went to the leaders and said, "Go on; blow off. We bought this land and it has been zoned for these houses and we're gonna build them. If you don't like it, that's your problem. Just get lost." She cut them no slack.

But it doesn't always work. In Miami there was a for-profit developer who wanted the same land as Habitat, and he went around and stirred up the neighbors. He fed their fears by saying all these new home owners were prostitutes, muggers, robbers, or thieves. The Habitat people thought, rather naively, that if they talked to the neighbors, they'd be able to convince them, so they called a big rally on a Sunday afternoon. The people all came, and Geoff Springer, the president of Miami Habitat, stepped up to the microphone to begin to talk. Even before he could say one word, a big guy jumped out of the crowd and ran right up and hit him in the face with his fist saying, "Get out of our neighborhood; we don't want you here." So they were never able to say a word, and the frightened Habitat for Humanity people gave up and never built there. They just went to another neighborhood.

I would say that what we are trying to do in Habitat for Humanity is to incarnate God's love. Love changes things; it is the most powerful force in the world. A person motivated by love is the most potent force there is. There are other forces that are potent, such as hatred. But love is a greater force. And what we are trying to do, in a very practical way, is unleash the power of love through the simple act of building houses. In the process, people come to appreciate one another. And it enables them to have a new understanding of what it means to be religious, what it means to be an authentic Christian, someone who has incorporated the principles and ideas of Jesus into her or his life, so they become a natural part of who the person is.

At the time when I was in turmoil because my wife had left me, I saw a movie on television. A young Chinese military officer had fallen in love with a woman missionary, and he was in a dilemma because he wanted to marry this woman but he knew that if he did, it would ruin his career in the Chinese army. So he went to a village leader, an old Mandarin, and posed his problem to him; the Mandarin responded by saying that a planned life can only be endured. This deeply affected me. Somebody once said that so many people tiptoe through life hoping to arrive safely at death, fearful of leaving a job they detest because of their pension plan. I think a person who does that is not living but enduring.

To live an unplanned life, you have to step out in faith. You either trust God or you don't. And trusting God is scary, because what if He's not there? I think that stops a lot of people: "I'd like to trust God, but what if I take a step off the cliff and I crash to the bottom?" That holds people back. But what I say is to take the step, for faith by definition is something you cannot prove; you just have to do it. And you have to be willing to fall on your face. I think that's a wonderful, incredibly exciting way to live. And you are willing even to suffer ridicule or misunderstanding to experience that kind of life. One of the most satisfying feelings you can ever get in life is that you're part of something that is making a difference.

Dr. A. T. Ariyaratne

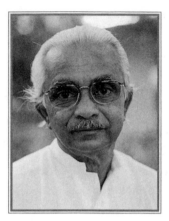

ounder of the world's largest movement for social change, the Sarvodaya Shramadana Movement in Sri Lanka, Dr. A. T. Ariyaratne has empowered thousands of people through his vision of the "awakening of all through sharing." "Whatever the global problems we have," he says, "they can be tackled satisfactorily when loving and selfless qualities are nourished and strengthened."

A New Social Order

It is my belief that we should courageously go beyond the narrow confines of conventional concepts and practices of social work and get to the roots of global sickness with a commitment to finding lasting remedies. After many years of working with and for people and learning from them, I have confidence in only one view. That is of people organized together as families and as small communities acting as advocates of their true interests.

As I grew up, I knew very little about Mahatma Gandhi's teachings, but on February 1, 1948, I saw a crowd of people in my village peeping at a newspaper and crying aloud as if a national calamity had occurred. This unforgettable experience of his assassination stirred me to read whatever material written by him I could find.

From that young age of a midteenager I felt drawn to the Gandhian fold, to serving my village community, and to seeing for myself the conditions under which the poorest and most neglected communities lived in the backwoods of Sri Lanka. At that time it seemed impossible to conceive of any nonviolent way that the injustices these people were subjected to could be rectified. It was only some years later, while in India attending a New World Education Fellowship conference, that I first heard the word *Sarvodaya,* a term coined by Mahatma Gandhi to describe a new social order which he envisioned as being very different from the capitalist or communist systems prevalent at that time. Literally, it means the "welfare of all." We have interpreted it as meaning the "awakening of all through sharing." It awoke in me the ideal to which I have dedicated my life.

Sarvodaya work in Sri Lanka started among small, socially ostracized communities and gradually developed, gathering experience, almost as an "experiment in life," as Gandhi said. The Sarvodaya Shramadana Movement has been active for over forty years in the empowerment of the poor and the total nonviolent transformation of society, from the individual to the family to the village community, extending to the national and even the global community. This is a people's movement. Our entire philosophy is based on finding the weakest, most-underprivileged, powerless, downtrodden communities. Now we work in more than half the country's villages.

Sharing signifies a sense of community. In sharing there is no giver or receiver, and so egoism and pride or feelings of inferiority are avoided. In the practice of sharing, the dignity and respect of all human beings are given equal recognition. The forms of sharing may vary: one may share wealth, land, or other material resources with those who have less; another may share skills, knowledge, or labor. The development of loving-kindness toward all living beings and the sharing of compassion can be cultivated by all people.

Sharing can extend from one individual to another, between families and villages, and from there to the urban, national, and international communities. Sarvodaya has practiced the principle of sharing by bringing together tens of thousands of people within Sri Lanka and from other countries to build a "no-poverty, no-affluence" society. The methods used are nonviolent, constructive, self-reliant, and participatory. We define development as an awakening process that takes place in the spiritual, moral, cultural, social, economic, and political dimensions of human beings, in the family and in rural and urban communities. The object is to create a society in which every individual, family, and community is awakened to a more fulfilled, peaceful, and just life.

Firstly, we help the village community to come together at a psychological level, so the members can begin to feel as though they are part of one large family. This happens when they share their time and effort to perform a task that benefits them all. We select and discuss a useful task to be done together—with both villagers and volunteers from Sarvodaya—that will satisfy a real need of the community. Together we plan the project in such a way that everyone feels that he or she is engaged in the noblest task that any human being can conceive of: building a truly human society in which nothing but the best manifests itself. The shared task may be an access road to the village, a series of wells for clean water, an irrigation canal to the fields, or a building for a school and community meetings.

All the volunteers and the villagers—the men, women, and children—camp together for the time it takes to do the shared task. They cook, eat, clean, work, meditate, sing, and dance together, learning from one another without being formally taught. There is something more than road building or irrigation canals happening in these camps, something more than even what is now called human resource development. A continuing process of human personality awakening is released in this initial activity in the village; a respect for life prevails, a tolerance of cultural or religious differences, a compassionate service, and the joy one gains from such selfless service. We call this spiritual and psychological infrastructure building, an entirely different kind of psychological security mutuality founded on spiritual awakening.

We are one of the largest self-development groups in Asia,

but we do not spoon-feed people. We motivate them for self-reliance and community participation, showing them that, collectively, they have considerable resources to change their living conditions.

From the initial camps with volunteers, the second stage continues with the formation of groups of children, mothers, farmers, and so on. We work with the community leaders, providing appropriate technical training to develop their skills. This is known as the social infrastructure and leadership development stage.

In the third stage a representative village organization is formed and we assist it in becoming a legal, independent institution recognized by government agencies. Different committees take over responsibilities for different activities, such as conservation and improvement of the environment, health and education, and spiritual development and interreligious cooperation. Independent specialist institutions are set up from which village societies can draw knowledge, skills, and technical help and even get access to outside capital, loans, or grants. We help them with mobilizing their savings and generating credit programs and by financing microcredit enterprises through the Economic Enterprises Development Services of the movement.

The fourth stage is when they have their own organization, know-how, relevant technology, and finances and can sustain themselves as they proceed toward self-development, self-government, and self-sufficiency. They begin to take their future into their own hands.

The fifth stage is when the village leaders help nine other villages in their vicinity to develop their potential for self-development. Ten villages work together as a cluster. These clusters are coordinated as divisions in districts and on national levels so that there is maximum freedom and highest coordination toward achieving the Sarvodaya objectives. Such clusters multiply horizontally within the country, with international linkages. There are twenty-five districts in Sri

Lanka, and we have thirty-five district offices and three hundred and forty organizational centers. Over 11,300 villages out of an estimated 25,000 in Sri Lanka have organized themselves into village societies. This makes us a great challenge to the government. A past president said, "You are a government within a government, only ours is ruled by law and punishment and yours is ruled by moral values."

Balanced development includes many different aspects of society. That is why we operate a wide variety of programs, including drug abuse rehabilitation, human rights protection, AIDS education, and counseling for victims of civil war. We are affiliated with over five thousand preschools, and we have twenty orphanages, homes for the elderly and the disabled, management training centers, fifty centers working in the city slums, engineering workshops, and so on. Other programs include peace education and conflict resolution.

I believe no problem is caused by an isolated reason; every problem is related to so many other problems. No incident, however cruel, is separate from other social incidents, whether personal violence, organized crime, conflict, or war. Only an integrated approach to the problem will be a solution in both the short term and the long term. Human consciousness has to be raised to inspire greater loving-kindness and compassionate action. When there is greater awareness, crimes on children, sexual abuse, violation of human rights, and so on, can all be brought under control. Of course, intervention by the state will always be there, but we can reduce this to a minimum and instead generate people's power through spiritual and moral advancement, and develop a kinder and more-caring society. That is why Sarvodaya takes into consideration spiritual, moral, and cultural needs as well as social, economic, and political factors and develops an integrated program to assist the human personality, the family, and the urban and rural communities in a total awakening process. It is a force of social transformation.

There is a tremendous need for such social transformation in every part of the world. However, each individual must decide his or her own priority of action or path of service. This means developing a very personal spiritual goal as the motivating force; no action is worthwhile if the activist is not motivated by loving-kindness, compassion, and the dispassionate joy of service. To be a social activist is meaningless unless the activist undergoes a spiritual transformation, a reducing of anger and greed and an awakening of the personality. The success of a social activist, in my opinion, is proportional to the degree to which the inner defilements are cleansed in the process of being engaged in worthwhile social action. Then true transformation is possible.

Change does not always come easily; there can be many conflicts and misunderstandings to overcome. Due to uprisings in the late 1980s—in which one hundred thousand people died—and growing confrontation with the established order, I became the primary target of a hate campaign in the media and received many anonymous death threats. These conflicts strengthened the movement internally, and they gave us unprecedented public sympathy as a people's movement that not even a powerful government could stop.

It also taught me how to consciously extend loving-kindness and compassion to everybody I see and whoever comes to my mind, including those who insult me or want to destroy me. I maintain a state of mind that does not alienate me from other human beings but does keep away ill will and fear. This helps me to maintain a clarity of vision. I try my utmost to be peaceful within myself, and therefore I recognize no enemies. Anybody is free to be jealous of what I am doing or to hate me, but I do not treat them in the same way. I respond with love and forgiveness. Some call this a great weakness; I think it is my greatest strength. I do what I can to stop the insanity in the world, but the real thing is the sanity within myself.

Nobody can hurt or abuse you if you are aware and hold love in your heart. When you hear some bad words, just think "Words . . . words . . . words" and do not give meaning to the words by thinking "I am being abused." When someone creates sounds, it is the listener who gives the meaning of praise or abuse to those sounds. When our minds are trained to look at both praise and abuse as just a flow of sound without preference or meaning, then we can live in equanimity. If we allow everything to enter into our consciousnesses without discrimination, then we will suffer.

Ultimately compassion, cooperation, equanimity, morality, forgiveness, and selflessness are most effectively practiced in small communities; they cannot be centralized or manifested through large structures. What Sarvodaya is trying to do is to develop such communities and link them together, nationally and globally. A number of international movements have already flowered from this work in many different countries. They combine with other movements that have similar ideals in the formation of a critical mass of spiritual and psychological consciousness at the global level.

I believe that all political and economic structures should be restructured on a basis of human-centered social and community organizations in order to create a better world. Whatever the global problems we have—ranging from separation of human beings from one another to environmental degradation—they can be tackled satisfactorily when loving and selfless qualities are nourished and strengthened. It is in such a global society that the awakening or well-being of all will best be ensured.

If other countries can follow this kind of ideal, then the twenty-first century will be in the hands of people who have no ambition to rule over others or amass wealth just to satisfy their senses. They will live a peaceful and sustainable pattern of life. We must overcome our greed for power and wealth, master our own minds to establish self-governing communities, and learn the joy of living. We may take courage from what Mahatma Gandhi wrote to Shri Nehru more than a half-century ago: "The essence of what I have said is that man should rest content with what are his real needs and become self-sufficient. If he does not have this control, he cannot save himself. After all, the world is made up of individuals just as it is the drops that constitute the ocean."

Cathrine Sneed

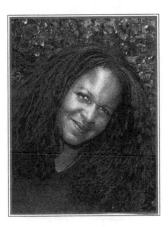

Her own illness inspired Cathrine Sneed, a jail counselor for the San Francisco Sheriff's Department, to get the inmates outside and working on the land. Since then, the Garden Project has provided work, motivation, and direction for thousands of prisoners and former prisoners. As she shares the story of the garden, she says, "I feel the garden gives people support and care. . . . Through the garden they find their human dignity and self-worth."

The Garden Project

Growing Urban Communities

I've worked for the San Francisco Sheriff's Department for eighteen years. When I first started working there, I was a counselor doing legal work with the women prisoners. Most of them were there for prostitution or petty theft; many were young mothers who had been in and out of jail over a period of years. They were basically poor women who hadn't finished school, didn't have any work experience, and felt they didn't have an alternative to prostitution or theft.

When I started, I was very excited to help these women because I felt that if they had access to legal services and someone to encourage them, they could put their lives in order. After a couple of years I began to see it was far more complicated than that. Even if they were able to get a restraining order to prevent their boyfriends or husbands from harassing them or making them get involved in crime, still most of them had no homes, no support, and children who were in foster care or with their parents. It wasn't just that they couldn't get a job. I would help them with divorces and restraining orders, as well as to get jobs wherever possible. I would get donations of clothes and toys and household goods and help them find housing.

But still that wasn't enough; they would come back to the jail, often in worse shape than when they had left. Due to the regular meals in jail, most of them gained weight there and began to look healthy, and then we threw them out of jail. At that time when prisoners were released, the county jail gave them a one-way bus ticket, which was about 85 cents, and that was all they left with. Sometimes they left wearing jail clothes because they had come in hot pants or high heels but they couldn't fit into those clothes anymore.

I saw the effect of being in jail on the women. A jail is a very noisy place, where everyone is talking, the television is on loud, some people are on the phone screaming so the other person can hear them, and the guards are walking around with these giant keys and they're screaming at each other, and then a fight will break out. It is very much what hell must be like. My job was to sit in a little corner with the women and listen to them and try to sort out what I could do and how I could help them.

In some cases they would have left their children with a pimp and they would ask me to go and find their children and try to get them away from the pimp and to their family members. Sometimes the children had been left in a hotel room by themselves, and sometimes the children ended up at home with my children for months at a time.

I believe it was being exposed to this hell for two years that made me develop a kidney disease, and I ended up in and out of the hospital for a couple of years. My doctor said they had tried all the treatments they could and that this disease was not treatable. So what more could they do? My doctor said, "You can stay here in the hospital and die or you can go home; it's your choice." That same day one of the people who came to visit me was the person who had convinced the San Francisco sheriff to give me my job. Ray had started education programs for prisoners of the jail. Before that the prisoners were just locked up and forgotten. He was a real innovator and also a real character. Ray gave me a copy of *The Grapes of Wrath* to read. He sort of threw it at me and said, "While you are sitting here dying, or thinking you are dying, why don't you do something like read a book? It's a powerful book, so read it. A powerful writer wrote it."

So I started reading the book and it grabbed me. I felt the story was clearly saying if people without hope and without future could connect with the land, they would somehow be able to overcome some of the obstacles, some of the problems, in their lives. Our jail is on 145 acres. In 1934 when the jail was built, it was a farm and the idea was to have the prisoners work on the farm. But over the years the farming had stopped and the sheriff's department had turned it into a storage place for old jail beds, old windows, papers, and furniture. An incredible valley was overcome with weeds and junk. While I was reading the book, I thought the answer was to bring the prisoners outside from the jail, so at least they could get out of their horrible rooms. At the time I didn't think of gardening as the thing to do; I just wanted to get them outside because as a kid I really liked being outside and thought it would be beneficial for them.

I said I was going home from the hospital and I wanted to go back to work and I wanted to bring the women prisoners out to the land. I was told that first I had to get better. I said I'm coming back to work now and I'd like to do this now. And I did. When I got back to work, I couldn't walk. I was in bad shape, and the prisoners were sad because of the way I looked. I had gone from being healthy and able to help them to being someone who couldn't even walk. I was impressed that they felt pain for me; I had never seen them feel pain for anything. The staff thought that the prisoners would hurt me if they allowed them to go out with me or that they would run away.

Well, what happened was when we started going out everyday, they literally carried me about half a mile down the road to this old farm and then they started cleaning up the mess, and they started to be very excited and caring about what we were doing. They were extremely gentle and caring about me. They never hurt me. After about a year we had a long waiting list of men who also wanted to get into the program, and slowly we started letting them in too. At one point we had maybe two hundred people on the waiting list and maybe sixty or so people in the program out there with the cleanup.

After about two years the disease went into remission and I started to get better. My doctor claims it was the chemotherapy, while I believe it was seeing this incredible transformation in the people I was working with. At the time a good friend of mine who is a gardener and a horticultural therapist came to work with us. She started by growing a small herb garden that we slowly expanded to vegetables. The prisoners were so enthusiastic about this. The vegetables we grew we took to the soup kitchens, to the homeless shelters, to senior centers. It was important that the prisoners had this opportunity to give because their whole lives had been ones of failure in which they were always taking and hurting others and never got a chance to be the good guys. They were excited about the amount of food that they were growing but also excited that they were now the good guys.

I remember one of the prisoners. His history had been one of assaults, mainly on seniors, and here we were giving the vegetables to the senior centers. I remember him saying, "My career was to hurt and take the purses of older women because they were vulnerable. I don't think I can do that anymore because I never thought of them as people and now I think of them as people and that has changed for me." You could see in this man's face that he was saying something that was true for him. The prisoners had found an activity that meant something, that gave them a sense of purpose.

Well, soon after the program began to develop, my friend the gardener had to leave, and so there I was with this garden and I knew nothing about gardening! So I got six months leave from the sheriff's department and began learning about growing food, and I developed a real appreciation and understanding of plants. I learned how to communicate my enthusiasm to the prisoners. We had classes every day and you could hear a pin drop. Here were people who had not finished school, who could barely read or write, but they would try to figure out what I was talking about. My enthusiasm about the plants infected them. Soon we were feeding all the soup kitchens in San Francisco. We were feeding about 1,200 people a week with produce from our garden, from the farm.

We had to fence in an area of about eight acres because we had a lot of deer that would come in. Now remember, these were people who were living behind bars because they constantly hurt people and sold drugs and did terrible things. And they didn't realize that deer were wild animals, so they would leave the gate open because they wanted the deer to be able to eat the lettuce. They would leave food for them and water for them! One time we had chickens and some skunks build their nest underneath our chicken coop. One day I came in and the staff was all upset. I thought something horrible had happened—a death, a fight, or something. What had happened was some of the men had noticed that some of the skunks underneath the chicken coop were babies. They thought they were cats. And what they did was move the chicken coop and carry these babies away. Of course, they got sprayed all over, and the staff got sprayed too. But what touched me most was that one of the prisoners was Frederick. He had had forty-one arrests mostly for violent offenses, and here he was making sure the skunks were moved to a safe place. I believe that gardening gives the prisoners a way to learn to express care.

Last year we took pumpkins to a kindergarten class of very poor kids. The teacher said, "Put the pumpkins here, and we'll sort them out for the kids while they sleep." When the kids woke up, they jumped up and down, screamed, and shrieked, they were so happy. The prisoners that had helped me bring the pumpkins saw the joy that those children had from those pumpkins; this one guy, I swear he had tears in his eyes because I'm sure he had never seen such joy before. He also felt, I think, how he had helped make that happen.

It's been about ten years since we started. We now have several different programs. One is still where the prisoners are working at the jail. They are also doing landscaping. There used to be a playing field behind the main jail, which houses nine hundred people, and the prisoners got out about an hour a week on this playing field. They would go out in groups of about one hundred. The playing field had never been properly paved. So frequently people were hurt and would end up in the hospital, or the authorities would close the yard down and they wouldn't even get that one hour out there. Now a class of prisoners meets each day and they're learning basic landscaping. They've landscaped this field. They are building a track and a football field. And they have planted flowers all over the jail; they've made a place where the staff can sit with flowers outside. And of course the deer eat them all!

To me the best part of the program is we now employ people after they've left the jail. I was beginning to hear from recently released prisoners that they would rather be in jail than be at home, which is awful. For most of them being in jail meant being in this program, and that was far better than their life on the street.

It was difficult to start the second part of this program. I would go to businesspeople and ask for donations and ask for help for the ex-prisoners. I would try to get the ex-prisoners jobs in landscaping. We had some success. But again I kept seeing former prisoners returning to the jail and being very happy to be there. Then a man said he happened to have a garbage dump behind his bakery. He suggested we put a garden there. When I first saw it, I was not very excited. For a few days I felt it was too big an undertaking. But I kept getting calls from people who wanted to come back to the jail to be in the program.

When we built the garden, I could only spend from four o'clock in the afternoon until it got dark with the people who would come. I wasn't paying them but I did get donations of food and clothes. I would get a few bus tokens for them. It took about two years to clean the garbage dump out and make this beautiful garden. Then I began to see that it was necessary for the people to be paid a wage because otherwise they would go back to selling drugs as most of them were doing that to basically survive. I needed to be able to compete with drug dealing, and the only way to do that was to pay a wage. I have two deputy sheriffs and a board of directors who have raised some money, and we spend about sixteen hours a day in the garden trying to grow as much as we can so we can sell it.

What is wonderful for me is that every day the people come from wherever it is they live; they come to work in the garden. Some of them live in the street. There's a young man, Philip, who is sleeping in our toolshed every night. The other day I saw him go out the gate and then climb back over the fence and go into the toolshed. I said, "Philip, I'm worried that there's no heat in this place, no hot water, and it gets cold." He said, "It's better than living with my family in the housing project, because everyone is using drugs and I don't want to be there." They live in the hotels and the housing projects. I had another young man who used to live in his car in the parking lot.

This program has now employed about six hundred people. They are paid six dollars an hour to start, and it goes up to eight dollars an hour. We sell the produce to restaurants, we sell it at farmers' markets, we sell it at churches on Sunday. Frederick is our number-one student. He's the one who moved the skunk babies. My sister was telling me that she had to stop Frederick at the farmers' market from fluffing the lettuce to make it look nice because it was getting bruised. People would come by and say, "Your table is so beautiful," and Frederick would fluff the lettuce. Frederick's criminal history is so terrible, and now he's responding to strangers who tell him his lettuce is wonderful. We begin at 6 A.M. but Frederick is there at a quarter to six. He is staying in a housing project that is being threatened with closure. I know from statistics what happens in that housing project; it has the most crime of any part of the city—all the stuff that Frederick has to literally walk over to come and fluff the lettuce. I think it's a kind of miracle. My new ploy with the fund-raising that we are constantly having to do is to have wealthy people come to the project, and then Frederick walks them the length of this eight-acre garden. He shows them every corner of the compost and every vegetable that he's planted. By the end of the tour they write the check, so it's very effective!

I realized that however successful it was, the participants were only in the garden from nine to five each day. Afterward they went home, and who knew what was happening there. I tried to identify those factors that would contribute to their rearrest to begin to deal with them. I decided to require that they also go to school or that they see their probation officers. I felt strongly that what was missing was the structure that you and I take for granted. No matter how enthusiastic Frederick is about the lettuce, he still needs to be able to read and write. And so I said to the guys, "If you want a paycheck, you have to go to school. You've got to go to our local community college and take college courses. You've got to get a bank account. You've got to see that probation officer. You've got to get a driver's license. I don't care if you've been driving all your life; you need a license."

The miracle for me is that all the participants are now going to school. They bring the registration papers, the class attendance sheets. Because most of them have addiction issues, I also said they had to get counseling. And the good thing is that here they get to talk with people who are no longer using drugs, people who are struggling to overcome their addictions. To me it is so amazing that they are doing all this stuff. George is a forty-eight-year-old who has been in state prison and is also HIV positive. A couple of weeks ago Michael Hennessy, the sheriff, came for lunch at the garden, and when Michael walked in the gate, George rushed over to him, pulled out his driver's license, and shoved it in his face. "Look at this," he said. "I'm forty-eight years old and I've been driving since I was nine and this is the first time I've had a driver's license." He was so happy.

People come daily begging me for a job. It's the hardest thing to say no. Particularly to the men who are older than I am, who have tears in their eyes, begging me for a job that pays less than eight dollars an hour. I've developed an elaborate way of not having to say no. I put them on a waiting list and tell them if they want to move up the list, they have got to be in school and get a driver's license.

Most of them have been drug dealers. They're not dealing drugs out there with calculators; they're doing it all in their heads. They're cutting grams, making change; they're really gifted that way. At the farmers' market, David, who mostly sold marijuana, can weigh out spinach and make change all in his head. People come and line up around our table, and David is getting the change going and moving it and he has it all under control. And his only other experience is selling marijuana!

Richard is a deputy sheriff who is assigned to work with us. He had worked in the jail for eleven years with the maximum folks, the most dangerous, the most aggressive, the most violent. I think he is about thirty-six, and he's been at the jail since he was in his early twenties. When I first started working for the sheriff's department, I came in and talked with the prisoners, and as far as I was concerned, the deputies—the guards—were the bad guys. But when Richard came to work with us, it was the first time I had an opportunity to really hear what happens with the guards. A jail is not a solution to crime, because not only does it destroy the human being who is the prisoner, it also destroys the human being who is the guard. Richard has never been married. When I asked him why not, he said, "It doesn't last because after you've been in the jail all day and when you go home, you can't come down. The wall you've built up doesn't come down. All the stuff you see makes you wonder about people and you can't trust them, and so you are not trusting."

Another part of the program is a Tree Corps program that involves us in planting trees for the city of San Francisco. We started it very slowly, planting trees in areas where they had problems with vandalism or theft. We now plant and maintain all of San Francisco's trees. The department of public works, I'm sure, didn't think we could be so successful at planting the trees. But what they began to see was that when we planted the trees, they were not vandalized or stolen. I think that's because everyone knows who is planting the trees.

Romaldo came to our program when he was fifty-one, and he had never had a job in his life. He had been a heroin addict for thirty years; his wife had been a prostitute to support their habit. When his wife got out of the jail, she begged me to hire her. And then a couple of days later Romaldo got out of state prison for the hundredth time and she brought him to the garden. He was still very angry and closed, so I was not inclined to hire him. Because I had known Maria was supporting this guy through prostitution, he was not one of my top choices. But she begged me to please hire him; she wanted him to get a chance. So I said, "OK, he's hired, but if he misses one day, if there's any problem, if he disrespects you, he's out and you can't even talk to me about it. I don't want any mess from him."

When Romaldo came, he started working by himself, mostly in the garden. Anything you told him to do he would do right away. He went from our garden program to helping us initiate the Tree Corps program. He taught himself to read and write by reading about trees and learning what the trees needed. He has three children that he and Maria didn't raise because they were back and forth from jail so much that the kids sort of raised themselves, and now they are also in jail. But they have grandchildren. Romaldo would bring his grandchildren to see the trees. And I think what Romaldo was saying was, "You know I didn't raise your parents good and I've been a really terrible guy, but look at these trees that I'm now planting. Look what I'm doing now."

When Romaldo was planting those trees, no one messed with them because Romaldo was one of the higher-level Mexican mafia members in prison. He had a really tough reputation. No one messed with Romaldo's trees. But I think the other thing with Romaldo's planting the trees is that when his peers saw him in the Mission District or in Bay View or on Army Street planting trees, the message got through that they didn't have to deal drugs. They didn't have to throw away their lives, because if Romaldo could make it, they could make it.

Romaldo has just gotten a job working for the bakery. He's responsible for all their deliveries. He has graduated from the GED program, the high school equivalency program. Maria helped him to learn how to read and write. They both have driver's licenses. They're moving into a two-bedroom apartment because there they can keep their grandchildren. I think the fact that I gave Romaldo a chance really affected him. I see him driving these big trucks. I'm very proud of Romaldo and Maria. I feel like their grandchildren won't have to go through what they went through. To me this is what this program is about. It's about helping the people to reach into themselves and get in touch with what is there already.

I have seen a lot of the schools in the neighborhoods where the people that go to our jail live. There's nothing living in these places. There's garbage, graffiti—places where children certainly shouldn't be. And so we started a school program for single mothers who are planting and maintaining gardens in some of the local schools. I heard from our participants that it makes them feel that they are somebody, that they can do something, because we took a garbage dump and made it into a garden or we took this school yard and made it into a beautiful place. We have this one school, Fred Hart, that had this huge sort of dust-bowl space. The dust was so bad they couldn't open the windows. We made it into an English perennial garden. It's a beautiful, beautiful space.

The last part of our program has been to expand our ability to meet the demands of restaurants. So what happens now is at the eight acres that was the garden for the prisoners at the jail, we bring in a van full of ex-prisoners to work each day. Ten years ago I would never have believed that the deputies would allow former prisoners to come back and work. It's wonderful and very funny because we roll up in this van every day, and the deputies know all the workers because they've all been in the jail before. There's supposed to be this elaborate procedure to get you in and out of the place, in which they check your driver's license, warrants, social security, and stuff. Now it's like they have forgotten about it. I think because they are so genuinely surprised to see these former prisoners coming to work every day. But also I think that they feel so hopeful to see these people alive and well.

With these added eight acres we plan to expand to the different farmers markets and to more restaurants and to try to be as self-sufficient as possible. We have people coming from all over the country to see what we are doing, to visit us and to see how to do it too. That's very exciting to me, that people will take our model and make it work in their community. I think this is how communities are built, very small, just one piece at a time. Our department of agriculture, the USDA, sent out a team of people to spend a few weeks with us, asking how did we do this. And now a manual is going to be distributed throughout the United States in fifty states, and it will be stamped USDA approved! I hope this can be a way to help people who are on welfare to get back to work, as well as ex-prisoners.

I feel the garden gives people support and care. That they are able to work and with their own hands grow something makes them feel so great in a way that nothing else could. It changes their lives. The garden helps to give people the strength to keep going. I believe that what draws people to it is the feeling that they are working as a part of a family in which everybody is lifting them up rather than putting them down. Through the garden they have found their human dignity and self-worth.

John Bird

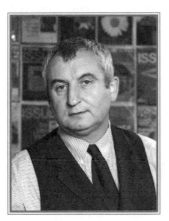

*F*ounder and editor-in-chief of the Big Issue *street magazine in London, John Bird has provided the means and incentive for hundreds of homeless people to rebuild their lives. A realist, he has a clear understanding of homelessness and poverty. "Homelessness is about social dislocation and a lack of motivation and the loss of meaning," he states. "With motivation you may not succeed but at least you are driven to get through the day."*

The Real Issue

I started the *Big Issue* as a street paper, because I had a friend whom I knew from the sixties who owned The Body Shop. He had seen a street newspaper in the United States, so he gave me the money. It started in 1991 to give homeless people an alternative to begging and a means to earn an income. It is a self-help initiative that offers a hand up, not a handout.

The *Big Issue* is sold by the homeless, ex-homeless, and vulnerably accommodated people. It provides an opportunity for people to help themselves by earning an income; vendors buy copies for 35p (50 cents) per copy and sell them to the public for 80p ($1.20). I wanted a street paper that was a good read and would give people an incentive to change. I didn't do it in order to lead a social transformation of the disgruntled and disenfranchised. I never realized it would become such a massive organization, but that only shows the need. It is now a magazine and we now have a circulation throughout Britain of upward of 300,000 issues a week. Most of our efforts go to helping people who are destitute, underperforming, not receiving help or support from anyone. We don't live in a perfect world, but we are doing what we can to help people who are in a social crisis.

Homelessness is not just about not having a home. It's about social dislocation and a lack of motivation. It's about the breakup of traditional things like industries in which people had jobs for centuries. It's about the increasing movement of people, the breakup of community, and the loss of meaning. The increase of crime on the street, drugs, and alcoholism are all signs of social instability. And I think that is the background from which homelessness becomes an expression of crisis. Homelessness is not a crisis in itself. If it were easy to solve homelessness by building more houses, then I would be a house builder. I'd be Britain's biggest property developer. Rather, I think the single biggest enemy to street people is lack of motivation, because with motivation you may not succeed but at least you are driven to face the next hurdle and to get through the day.

The *Big Issue* has addressed that central problem, that kernel of social collapse: the lack of motivation. It has given motivation to every vendor because it's up to them to make the magazine sell. I've never given to beggars; I give to performance. People who are putting effort into it, like a guy who was homeless for twenty years who has now, through selling the *Big Issue,* been able to create some stability in his life. Most homeless people have used it as a stepping-stone; when they get their acts together, they go away, and they don't always wave good-bye. Some of them do. I'll run into people who give me a whack on the back and say I used to sell the *Big Issue* and now I'm in advertising. There's a guy who is now a doorman, another who works at the BBC.

There are two things you shouldn't do to homeless people. One is to ignore them and the other is to sentimentalize them. You open your door to a homeless person and he or she will come in and rob you. It's not because I'm a cynic; I'm an optimist. But I've watched quite a number of homeless people. They say all the right things, and then you find something is missing, just because it's the kind of culture they are in in which everyone is out for her- or himself. It's also the problem of consistency. When I was in my twenties, I was inconsistent, I was a thief, I was doing all sorts of terrible things like I would rob my own girlfriends. I would know them for a few weeks and they would leave me in their house, and then when they came home, everything portable was gone. There is no honor when you've got your head up your ass.

A lot of people don't like that I'm a big mouth, that I'm like a secondhand car dealer. I'm not from the top drawer, and I'm certainly not somebody who is laden down with sociology degrees. Other people try to put me on a pedestal. Nobody is ideal; we wouldn't be in this vale of tears if it was so wonderful. But I've changed from how I was: I now pay on the train, I support my ex-wife, I support my children. If I'm on the train and somebody has his or her feet on a seat, I say put your feet down. A lot of the change came in me because I got involved in revolution and politics; I became a Marxist. I don't have a lot of time for Marxism now, but it got rid of a lot of the racist, xenophobic attitudes that you carry around when you come from the working class. It's very difficult to be a Marxist housebreaker or a Marxist racist.

How does the *Big Issue* help people? How are we helping people get their lives back together? By giving them an opportunity to work, to stand on their own two feet, to gain some self-esteem through self-help. We help homeless people largely by saying, "The greatest rejuvenation must come from within, not from without." The *Big Issue* gives people the opportunity to do things for themselves, from within, by making a commitment. You can turn someone around when you put her or him in front of the public; 80 percent of the rejuvenation is done out on the streets.

The Big Issue Foundation spends the profits of the *Big Issue* and other money that we raise. Selling the magazine is only the first step toward getting the homeless off the streets and into a stable place. People need help getting their lives together. So we help the vendors with support on the street, with safety and security and advice. We help them with housing problems, welfare rights, and how to cope when they do get housing, like how to cook or open a bank account. We teach them computer skills and secretarial and publishing skills and help them get an education. We have people offering emotional support and drug abuse counselors. When you've been on the street for five, ten, even fifteen years, you need help to get back in touch with how to do things. But you can do them, given the motivation. We do things like have poetry groups, art workshops, drama groups. We've had exhibitions and performances all over the country, all done by homeless people.

Don't accept the surface of things. Don't ever believe people can't be rejuvenated. Don't believe the world is made up of the good and the bad. I believe because you've done horrible things it doesn't mean to say, given the right kind of impetus and the right guidance, you could not be much better than somebody who has done it right all the time. A wonderful thing happens if you say to a homeless person, "We want you to help us. We need you to raise money for a children's hospital or to help a street paper in another part of the world." They jump at the chance to help because however abject they may be, they can help people who are more abject. It's a wonderful key. When I was in jail, I remember some of the nastiest people I had ever met being passionately involved with the stuffed toy class because they knew that those stuffed toys were going to be sold at an auction and that the money was going to go to the local hospital.

The first thing about powerlessness is a contract between the powerful and the powerless. If you work for me and moan about how nothing changes, then you are just a moaner and you have an unwritten contract that says you have given your power to me. You don't have to enter into that agreement. You don't have to enter into that agreement with the state, with the authorities, with business, or with individuals. It's a conscious decision to be worthless. You make the decision and you can renegotiate the contract.

How you do that is by doing very simple things like cleaning yourself up, thinking about what you are eating, thinking about how you relate to people. You do it by using things like libraries and public resources. In other words, you think about what you can put into the pot instead of what you can take out. You regain your power by renegotiating your power. It's not like somebody is there to renegotiate it. If you don't rise again, you've accepted the contract; you are saying I've lost. I think a lot of homeless people could be socially very useful, in the sense of being a poacher turned gamekeeper. I'm a poacher turned gamekeeper. You've got to get into the mind of the poacher in order to make the change.

Homelessness has become the pimple on the face; it's the form, not the content, of the social problem. The content of the social problem is the dislocation from society. I think one of the reasons why motivation has gone out of so many people is probably historic. Up to the mid-1930s, everybody did what they were told. They didn't try to get out of their class or social grouping. And then World War II came along and a lot of that broke up. The creation of the new world made people healthier and to some extent better mentally and physically. But what it didn't do was replace the old community and the old sense of belonging. So what we've got now is this yawning gap, a cultural gap where people don't feel they belong anywhere. And they are right.

I think this is about consumerism and the growth of individualism; it's about materialism and having prosperity and signs of importance around you. I think the quest for competition has created so many neuroses. We are living in a century in which people are alienated from each other, obsessed with the inadequacies of their living. They have to aspire to a new lover, a new house, and so on.

One of the advantages of the development of the economic

worldview in the nineteenth century was that it gave people work and a sense of belonging. Now you have a growth of an underclass that really has no social role. In the Victorian period you had homeless people, thousands living on the streets of London and in the parks. But they had a social role. They worked at the gasworks; they worked on the docks. It was cheaper for the employers to have mass casual labor. So the homeless may not have been very happy living in the streets but they had a social purpose. Now they don't have a social purpose because the system doesn't need them anymore.

If everyone woke up tomorrow morning and said, "It's possible; whatever it is, it's possible," and spent a whole day having an "it's possible" day, then we would be going down the kind of road I'm interested in—because I do believe it is possible.

Glenys Kinnock

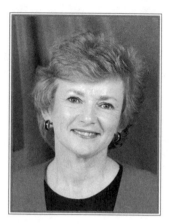

A politician at heart, married to the former U. K. Labour Party leader Neil Kinnock, Glenys Kinnock was elected as a Member of the European Parliament in 1994. Here she talks about One World Action, the developmental nongovernmental organization (NGO) of which she is president. "We have to recognize that there is a universal sense of responsibility that is called for," she says, "and we can't just give it out in small portions when it suits us. We have to absolutely believe in human rights and issues of equality; there is no halfway house."

One World

A great friend of mine, Bernt Carlsson, was the U.N. representative in Namibia when he was killed in the Lockerbie plane crash. Bernt was traveling to New York with the proposal for the transition from apartheid to a peaceful election in Namibia. He was a man who spent his entire life working on international issues, so I thought it would be appropriate to establish a development agency working in Namibia in his memory. People said, "There are enough agencies. Why do you need another one?" but I felt that there was a need for an agency or a group of people working together with different perspectives on the eradication of poverty, with ideas of self-help through the identification of people's own priorities in their own communities.

One World Action doesn't have people based in the developing countries; we don't have Land Rovers and field officers and teams of people supervising the projects. We work directly with groups of people—trade unions, cooperatives, environmentalists, and women's groups—we identify with them what their needs and concerns are, and then we help fund them. It's all very carefully monitored but without the old-fashioned paternalistic approach to development.

The need is terrifying, especially when you look at the levels of poverty. But I'm not pessimistic about the possibility of achieving change. We believe in "bottom-up" development. We reject the idea that benefits will trickle down from successful, prosperous organizations to the very poorest. It is our objective to target directly the very poor people who are invariably voiceless in the situations in which they find themselves. Running alongside such direct funding is the understanding that our campaigning and advocacy work in the West, such as in the United Kingdom, is of equal importance. All our partners in the developing world want us to learn from our experience of working with them and then to translate that into messages for the industrialized nations, messages that show that there is a new definition of rights and that there are other perspectives we can have and arguments we can make.

I think that if you understand what your own environmental priorities are and your own human rights priorities, you will find it much easier to understand people in faraway places who assert the need for equal rights for themselves. When CNN turns up in Zaire or Rwanda or Sierra Leone, we get negative images of vulnerable, pathetic people standing in line for food or sitting in refugee camps looking completely despairing. But there are other, very positive images of hugely impressive things going on. Instead of fire fighting when crisis and conflict occur, we should be tackling the root causes of poverty and disadvantage in the developing world. And once we make that leap of imagination, then the chances of seeing such awful tragedies are far less.

My father was a merchant sailor, so from the age of thirteen he told me stories of what he had seen in the United States, Africa, and Russia—of the inequalities. He implanted in me an awareness of injustice. Children always understand the words "It's not fair," whether the words apply to them when they are not given an ice cream or are about something much bigger. In 1956, at the time of the Suez crisis, the general attitude in Britain tended to be that we should stand up for our rights against Nasser and the Egyptians; but the message I got at my home was, "No, the canal belongs to them. It's theirs, and they're quite right to claim it for themselves."

I'm always deeply affected by what I experience. I vary between being very angry about the injustices and feeling very sad, especially when I see desperately poor people who have very little control over their own futures, who are unable to give their kids food or provide them with school uniforms or vaccinations, things that any normal parents want to do for their children.

What I always know is that I get on an airplane at the end of my stay; I go back to my comfortable life, while they have to continue grappling with enormous hardship. That's really what galvanizes me to want to raise awareness. Awareness is the most important thing, because all that is lacking is political will. There's no reason not to address all these problems, but governments, politicians, and financial institutions have to be motivated to do it. They could transform all those people's lives. We have to keep banging on the drum in the hope that they will pay attention.

Two of the major influences for change are the World Bank and the International Monetary Fund. If they are prepared to tackle the debt problem, then the many countries, particularly in Africa, that are spending more on repaying debts than on health and education could start to look after their people. We require the financial and the transnational companies to change their ways to a sense of responsibility toward the people they deal with, the countries and the communities that they affect. This would transform thousands of lives.

We have to protest very strongly against governments that are shortsighted, that don't seem to grasp the implications of what they do when they put trade before people. The most effective way to change policies is that the people who vote for the politicians demand that they change the way they behave when they are in office. We have to raise awareness about the inequalities between North and

South (developed and developing countries). People need to be urged to put pressure on their members of Parliament, their representatives and senators, in order to make them wake up to change, to the fact that it doesn't have to be like this.

Unless we tackle the implications of poverty, we will suffer the repercussions. We can't escape this; poverty is ticking away out there like a bomb, and it'll explode in all our faces if we don't deal with it. A billion people living in absolute poverty, so they don't know where their next meal is coming from, is like a boomerang. It doesn't need a passport to travel to other parts of the world. Whether through migration, environmental pollution, growth in the narcotics trade, or even internal terrorism, there is a multitude of impacts that we will suffer from if we don't tackle poverty at its source.

Everything is linked; the world is interconnected through technologies, communications, and especially trade. Those who are dealing with the impact of globalization tend to become paralyzed by the very word, incapable of saying that we can challenge its effects. But the beneficiaries of globalization have not been the poor people but transnational companies. So we need to reexamine our relationship with the World Trade Organization and challenge the view that liberalization, privatization, or other panaceas are the answer. In my view they are undermining much of the work that needs to be done to ensure greater equality in different parts of the world. Trade is terribly important but it must not always override principle. When it comes to dealing with countries where there is a flagrant abuse of human rights, without good governance or respect for people's rights, then we should be stepping back and saying, "Do we want to deal with these people?"

We need to think very carefully about how we respond. There are many countries across the world where I would like to see us taking much stronger action, such as economic sanctions, because that's the only thing these repressive regimes understand. They don't deserve pleasantries, because pleasantries are not what they use to deal with their own people, so they wouldn't understand them from us.

Education provides information to people so that they can make their own judgments. Look at the way we can decide on what to buy in supermarkets on the basis of how and where it has been produced. People are saying that they want to buy "solidarity" coffee or tea. They want to know from their supermarket whether the beans or the fruit that they buy have been produced where the people have got decent working conditions. When they buy a rug, people are asking, "Has it got a mark on it that says children haven't been used to produce it?" These pressures are increasing. We are learning that what we do actually results in successful outcomes.

All that is missing is common justice, nothing else. I don't feel at all depressed or pessimistic, because people are so fantastically strong and resourceful. Everything that we do should be pro-poor, should be targeted at ensuring that we eradicate poverty from the world. I believe that is an achievable objective. Everything can be solved, and we owe it to the people who are battling just to survive. There is no time to be saying it's just hopeless or to wring our hands in despair and give up on all this. We have no right to do that. The only option is to affect policies and create more awareness. It's not so long ago that it would have been unimaginable that someone from my working-class background could have gone to university and done the things that I and my kids have done. It is already a different world from the one that my grandparents or great-grandparents lived in. So enormous change is possible.

We have to recognize that there is a universal sense of responsibility that is called for, and we can't just give it out in small portions when it suits us. We have to absolutely believe in human rights and issues of equality; there is no halfway house. Gustav Speth of the United Nations said, "We have to work for equality, between nations, among nations and between women and men." That is what everyone who has the power to effect change should be working for, because if we don't share that objective, then we're not recognizing that we share a common future.

The nature of today's world is such that our futures are inseparable. A baby born last October somewhere in Africa, at the same time that my granddaughter was born in Brussels, is destined to have a completely different life with a completely different set of opportunities and options from my grandaughter's, from nutrition to education to health care and housing, just because of where she was born. My granddaughter will share a world with a baby born into desperate poverty in Africa or Asia. I would rather they have a shared future, one that doesn't reinforce the disadvantages but strengthens the connectedness.

Bo Lozoff

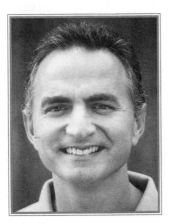

Through the Prison-Ashram Project, Bo Lozoff has reached thousands of prisoners in search of release from personal torment by encouraging them to use their limited conditions as a tool for inner freedom. "Either we are going to awaken to true compassion [for everyone], or we are not going to have compassion for anyone, even our loved ones . . . because love is love. You cannot turn it on and off like a water tap."

The Prison-Ashram Project

Growing up I had an uncle and two cousins in prison, and then my brother-in-law was involved in a drug deal and got a long sentence— twelve to forty years, five of them in a pretty grim institution. So I became conversant with the whole prison scene and began to wonder what we could do to help those inside. Sita, my wife, and I were living on an ashram (a Yoga community) when Ram Dass came to visit. He said he had started receiving mail from prisoners because he had donated copies of his book *Be Here Now* to all the prison libraries in the country, and would I be willing to deal with the correspondence? That was the beginning of the Prison-Ashram Project.

We were assuming that the people in prison who would be most interested in what we were offering would be doing time for manufacturing LSD or something kind of sophisticated and nonviolent. But during the first few years we were hearing from the rank-and-file prison population—low-education people who hurt or killed other people—and it was a big challenge. Then we had a visit from a safe cracker and ex-con, someone whom we had been with in the civil rights movement. He came to the ashram and asked me what we were doing. After I told him, he turned to me and said, "Bo, if you can't explain it to me the way I can understand it, then either it's not for real or you don't understand it." That hit me hard and made me realize that we had to really work on the simplicity of expressing spiritual truths. So we wrote *We're All Doing Time* as a way of reaching everyone, whatever his or her background. It is given free to any prisoner who asks for it, and now over 115,000 copies have been published.

Recently we went to death row at Central Prison, North Carolina. Here you have a bunch of condemned men who have no chance of getting out. I tell them that I am there in complete respect of them as human beings, with whatever beliefs they may hold, that I do not see them as just a compilation of their actions. Maybe no one has ever before treated them as real human beings, let alone as spiritual seekers, but that's how I see them. There is never anyone it's too late for. So I'm telling them they are not wasted, it's not too late to have genuine peace in their hearts. Most people do not know when they are going to die, whereas these men do know, so they can truly prepare themselves. And we talk about how death can be beautiful, how it can be a time of great liberation.

We're trying to make spiritual activists out of the prisoners we meet. We see them as reflective people, capable of great transformation. I don't think it is possible to get a happy life through crime or through trying to figure out a self-centered solution; I don't think it's about getting a master's degree while you are inside so you can make $50,000 a year when you get outside. Some of the prisoners do this and then find they are not getting the happiness they thought they would. I think the only viable option is to be dedicated to something larger than ourselves. To move from a life that is basically self-centered to one that is other-centered. This is a very powerful message for those who are tired enough of their selfish patterns, who have had enough of the violence and pain.

This guy who had murdered his girlfriend with an ax wrote to me and said he wanted to feel some peace. I responded by saying,

You did a terrible thing and you will experience the consequences of it for the rest of your life; you know that. But what you don't know is that life is solely and entirely a spiritual journey and that it is never too late to realize this. Even a life that seems a total waste can end up having a lasting meaning. Your crimes need not be wasted. In every religion there are stories of the poor, the thieves, or the murderers being saved. For whatever reasons that you did what you did, this is your path up the mountain. If you take a selfish path, you are basically just trying to make your pain go away. You will not find your way out of this through selfishness, but you will find meaning and purpose and strength by changing your lifelong patterns of selfishness. If you take a spiritual, unselfish path, you are going to gain compassion and wisdom. This will take a lot of practice and vigilance. That is what we are here for, all of us. Whether you are in prison or not, nothing is as important as feeling the grace of Divine love.

Devoting our lives to others is vital, but not just so we get to feel better. Everywhere we hear about the benefits of doing service. People are putting some volunteerism into their lives because it's supposed to make them happier; it has even become a cliché to say, "I get much more out of this than anyone I have ever helped." But this is debasing the motivation for service, making it a selfish act rather than a selfless one. Altruism—the act of doing something for the benefit of others—must itself be altruistic. Altruism is giving up the self, saying, "enough about me." Instead it's saying, "I don't know whether it's going to make me happy or not, but I've got to help those kids/AIDS babies/the environment/whatever, simply because they or it need help." When something pulls on your heart and you respond without any thought of yourself, then the results don't matter.

We've come up with so many rationalizations to encourage us to think about ourselves first, but it's not working and it's not going to work. I'm not saying we should pretend not to know that service is a time-honored path associated with deep peace and happiness. But we need to remember that it is not a path about our happiness; rather, it's a happy path. True selflessness is like a smile: it arises naturally in a life lived well. We don't stand in front of the mirror all day working on our smile, do we? Smiling is a natural part of life. So are self-esteem and personal happiness. They are impossible goals if pursued selfishly, yet they are free gifts when we give up self-absorption.

As we worked with the Prison-Ashram Project, the thing that struck us most was how similar prison life was to the ashram we were in. We woke up at 4 A.M., we wore white, we worked hard on the farm all day without being paid, we didn't go to the movies, we were celibate, we ate in groups, and we didn't snack between meals. And then we would go to visit my brother-in-law at the prison farm in Indiana. He was waking up at 5 A.M., and he was wearing all white, working on the farm all day without getting paid, not having sex (not that he would talk about anyway), eating in groups, and not snacking between meals. We were the ones that were free while he was in prison, yet we had elected to give up most of the pleasures and freedom of choice that he was dying to have. So it struck us that whether we are in a prison or an ashram, it is much the same; we are all doing time.

We all have our various forms of chains or limitations, so it seems that apart from discovering the spiritual nature of life, no matter what situation we are in, there is something inherently incomplete, a level of agitation or wanting, desiring, and being unsatisfied. We get so many letters from the families, friends, or social workers of people in prison saying that they feel just as locked up as the ones behind the bars. They share that they are not happy with their lives, that they feel unhappy or frustrated. This is the place where we are all doing time. The modern-day United States has made personal pride a great virtue instead of a dangerous vice. Pride is in, modesty is out; assertiveness is in, easygoing is out; boastfulness is in, humility is out; competitiveness is in, self-sacrifice is out. It's amazing that we keep presenting this same model of success to our kids, year after year, when there is so much evidence that the more we get of it, the sadder or more dysfunctional we become.

There's a wonderful reason that personal pride, self-esteem, boastfulness, and selfish success don't lead to happiness. The reason is this: we are all deeply connected. We are in this thing together from start to finish. We are one big family, like it or not. We need each other. We are one big event, all of us together, and we must either start acting like it or else descend further and further into despair, madness, or mass annihilation. Our society is terribly unhappy precisely because our true nature is divine and generous and merciful, but we're not acting like it. This means that we can wake up from this horrible national hangover we're experiencing. Enough of the arrogance and pride, of the "I Deserve Prosperity" seminars and the "Free Yourself from Guilt" workshops. Enough about "me" already! We need to look around and realize that we only exist in relation to each other.

Our true nature is compassion. We cannot be compassionate to our children or our parents or our spouses if we are not also compassionate to the guy who is guilty of multiple rapes or murders. Either we are going to awaken to true compassion or we are not going to have compassion for anyone, even our loved ones. If I don't love Charles Manson, then it means I'm not going to be able to really love my own son, because love is love. You cannot turn it on and off like a water tap. True love is a state of seeing clearly. If we choose to see clearly, then we have compassion, then we will love, and once we choose to really love, then we cannot exclude anyone. That would mean we are putting conditions on that love, which turns it into a whole different thing. It's not going to be real love unless it includes everything and everyone.

The problem is that we are told it is all right to be cruel and vicious to those who have harmed us, to celebrate when someone is executed, to hate our enemy. But it just doesn't work to sanction ill will, anger, or hatred, even when people have wronged us. This doesn't mean we condone terrible things, but when we see clearly, we see there is just one big self. Look at the Sermon on the Mount: two of the beatitudes are saying to love those who harm us, despise us, and persecute us. So this is not a new teaching—it goes back a long way—and its essence is not to cast anyone out of our hearts. We may have to lock them up, but we don't have to shut them out of our hearts. A spiritual truth that doesn't hold up in a prison cell or during an earthquake isn't a big enough truth. The big truths are true throughout any possible condition life can present to us.

When we choose faith, it doesn't mean that bad things no longer happen to us; it just means that there is no longer any cause for fear or bitterness in our pain. Fear is a powerful addiction; that's why it takes a while to develop the sort of faith that makes no room for fear. Fear says, "You'd better watch out; it's dark up ahead!" But with a daily practice of faith you can remind yourself, "Of course it's dark up ahead. Up ahead is not my business; this moment is, and it's light enough for me to see right now." We can be like a coal miner carrying his light on his cap. Wherever he arrives, it's light enough for him to see. He doesn't sit in one place and say, "But it's dark up ahead."

When faith replaces fear, there will still be sadness, sorrow, or grief in our lives, but they will be soft around the edges instead of hard. They will make our hearts bigger instead of closing them off to try to keep out further pain. An earthquake can humble us instead of terrify us. A setback from the parole board can sadden us instead of defeat us. Being HIV can inspire us to dig deeply into the preciousness of our remaining time here. When we have chosen to feel that we belong here in this world and that we are cared for by the loving intelligence that guides it, then we no longer feel like nameless insects victimized by a vast, chaotic universe which neither knows nor cares that we exist. Every place becomes our home, and every event works in our favor, no matter what it looks like to the world.

It just takes practice—a little ego risk and lots of practice. We start with shaky faith; now and then we feel some shaky peace. As we risk stronger faith, we occasionally feel stronger peace. When our faith becomes unwavering, our peace is constant and unshakable. If we consider the options (and there aren't any good ones I can think of), it's not a bad deal. It just takes practice.

So, why not give yourself a chance to find out for yourself whether all this is real or not? Be a spiritual practitioner for a month or two and see whether your life feels any different. It will never be fully convenient to begin. If you think you have to wait for something, you are missing the point, and you may well be waiting forever. Now is the only time we can ever use. I gave a guy in the Kansas State Prison a heart-centered meditation to do, and he wrote and told me how suddenly he felt like his whole heart cracked open. He looked around and saw how everything in the prison was exactly the same but it was glowing, just like how Christmas was meant to be when we were kids but never quite was. And he saw everyone doing the same old thing, but they were doing it so beautifully.

So how do we best help the world? For me, it comes down to just two things. Firstly, it is important to strive to do my best, to do impeccable work, no matter what the work is; and, secondly, I must strive to express kindness and goodwill through my thoughts, words, and deeds. And if I do just these two things, that's the most I can do to bring about any kind of betterment in the world. A project like the Prison-Ashram Project is mainly a means to encourage others to do the same, to strive hard at everything they do and to make sure their motivations are always to benefit others. The ideas and teachings from saints and sages are merely to reinforce these ideas; the practices we give are merely to enable the individual to put these two simple things into action. Dharma, or truth, can be stated in innumerable ways, but it boils down to personal effort and altruistic motivation.

The Prison-Ashram Project is our way of communicating Dharma to people who find themselves in dire circumstances, albeit one of the best and most classic seedbeds for deep transformation. We remind prisoners of saints such as Paul and Dismas in Christianity, Milarepa and Angulimala in Buddhism, Valmiki in Hinduism, and Bilal in Islam—all perfectly horrible and brutal people until they experienced great spiritual transformation, after which they became saints and prophets. We remind people that it is never too late, regardless of what they have done. There is no deed, however heinous, which we cannot use toward the perfection of our humility and compassion.

So we find ever-fresh ways of reminding people of these simple timeless truths, encouraging them to find and follow their own paths to sainthood. I don't imagine the prisons are now bursting with saints, but we have certainly seen great and sincere transformation which inspires us to continue this process of sharing and cajoling. In twenty-five years I have never yet met a person who did not want to be respected as good and decent. We are all the same in more ways than we are ever different. If we could remember this, then we wouldn't be thrown for such a loop when people present the many masks they wear, whether through fear or delusion. We merely look through those masks, as a parent would spot her or his own child behind a Halloween costume, and say, "Hello in there, dear one." And the dear one generally, even if slowly, emerges to return the greeting. An hour later that person may be back behind the mask as he or she moves about the prison, but hopefully he or she had a few minutes' relief from the playacting and will remember how good that felt. When ready to drop the mask entirely, the person will, just like the rest of us. We are holy, and we pretend we are not. It's the Great Mystery, isn't it?

Sulak Sivaraksa

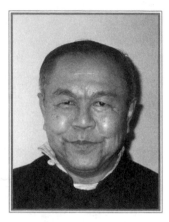

A revolutionary and social activist in Thailand, Sulak Sivaraksa has often confronted the Thai authorities in his quest for human rights and spiritual and social freedom. Tireless in his work to generate greater awareness and honesty on all levels, he says in his piece, "To care for our own community, we must think more of each other and of creating a compassionate way of life that does not bring pain."

Social Activism

Concern for human democracy, human rights, and accountable government has been the main thrust of my life and work. I am outspoken in my beliefs, and as a result, from time to time, I have had to go into exile because I could be arrested or my safety could not be guaranteed. I have been in jail as a consequence of my outspokenness against the Thai government and the way it treats the Thai people. In 1963 I founded the *Social Science Review*, which played a crucial role in stimulating student awareness prior to the 1973 uprising when the military regime was overthrown. The government has now come to realize that it must tolerate outspokenness, it must listen to the truth, and that what I and others have been trying to do through nonviolence is of great value. This year, army and police officers have come to study nonviolent techniques; this is wonderful.

I consider myself an engaged Buddhist, one who is involved with social activism from a Buddhist perspective. In traditional Buddhism we care for our own well-being—physical, mental, and spiritual—as well as the well-being of others, of society. Buddhism advocates, as a basic principle, nonviolence, or ahimsa. It is not easy to maintain an attitude of nonviolence when all around you there is rape, murder, and child abuse. We need more seeds of peace.

After 1988 many Burmese students were killed; others fled to the Thai border. They were full of violence. I made friends with them and built trust, and then I was able to offer them something skillful. We established the Jungle University for Burmese refugee students, so they could continue their education. Certainly they wanted to raise arms; they wanted to fight. But some have come to understand the nonviolent approach. To confront issues doesn't help. Twenty years ago many Thai students were killed; they were betrayed. Now many of them realize that the principle of ahimsa is very deep.

I feel that such consumerism and violence is dominating the world that we must be able to challenge this unjust social structure nonviolently, to become more indigenous, to care for our own community. We have developed many social welfare organizations in Thailand to help people in the way they need it. A lot of people question nonviolence and say that in some circumstances we have to be violent. Nelson Mandela has spoken of how he felt it becomes immoral to pursue a policy of nonviolence as it simply allows the suppressor to continue. To be honest, I cannot say that nonviolence is the only answer. But neither can I vouch for violence. For me, violence has a much worse outcome than nonviolence. I remember my U.S. Quaker friends who went to Hanoi during the Vietnam war, and the Vietnamese said to them, "How can we use nonviolence when you people are bombing us like this?" There is no answer to that. I simply could not be violent; it would go against everything in my being. Somebody may say it's escapism, but I could not justify it morally.

If we are limited in resources and time, how can we apply social activism? What things can we do that would have the greatest effect? I think change happens when we see somebody who is suffering; then I think we will change our lifestyle because we will see where we can be less materialistic, less of a consumer, where we can take less and give more. It is not right to accumulate wealth while people are homeless and suffering. We feel the more we acquire, the more we will be happy, but that is not the case. When we make our lifestyles more simple, we gain a greater happiness.

This means starting from our own insights. If we are peaceful, if we are harmonious with ourselves, then we will see things as they really are. If we don't have that insight, we are bound to be unskillful, to cause harm or hurt. There is an important teaching in the terms *skillful* and *unskillful*. If we are not clear in our vision, then what we do will ultimately be for our own egoistic needs. Many of us do things in the name of social justice, in the name of ideology, but unskillfully, without awareness or sensitivity. And that is bound to hurt both ourselves and others.

I have been involved in helping drug abusers to heal their lives, as well as working with AIDS patients. This has helped me personally, for when I am confronted with drug addicts, I am reminded of the impermanence of life. It reminds me that these are fellow sufferers, that we all suffer in life. So I do anything I can to help them. We feel that medicine alone does not help, especially with AIDS. Those who have AIDS need more to help them confront the suffering within themselves. So at the same time we use skillful means to show them how to be calm, how to meditate, how to find peace.

Forgiveness is very important. In order to forgive, we must cultivate fearlessness. When we are fearless, we can forgive, yet we are full of fear. We have to empower ourselves spiritually; otherwise we forgive only with our words. We can forgive an action with words, but it still remains in our hearts and our minds. If we really want to forgive, this is where deep meditation practice is essential. Aung San Suu Kyi was put under house arrest and she forgave her oppressor. She said, "I have no fear." It is the same with the Americans who went back to Vietnam to help their former enemies. Then forgiveness becomes beautiful. Then I think we become full human beings. I don't forgive that easily, especially governments, but one good thing about becoming old is eventually I do get to forgive. My wife says I have become much more effective now because I use less violent words! Although I have never been violent, I now use more and more beautiful words; I try to praise people rather than to blame them, to see what is right rather than what is wrong.

If I don't forgive, then it stays in me. Forgiveness is really selfish as you feel so much better when you forgive. Ultimately you must cultivate loving-kindness and compassion for others, for the enemy. Then you see how we are all interrelated.

I try to maintain certain times of the day to be quiet, to breathe, to feel forgiveness and compassion. As a Buddhist I hope eventually to reach Nirvana, but since I have not yet reached that ultimate, I try to reach Nirvana at least a few moments every day, to be peaceful, to be clear of all defilements. When you are involved in social activity, if you don't have peace of mind, then sometimes your egoistic tendency will come in. You are doing it because you want to be recognized. And sometimes also you get hurt because people blame you when things do not go well. So we have to be skillful, to be understanding and forgiving, to bring more compassion into our lives and into the world. We must think more of each other and of creating a compassionate way of life that does not bring pain.

My solution for change, for those who want to make a difference, is very simple. Everyone should spend at least five to ten minutes every day breathing deeply. I think that would make a huge difference, because breathing is the most important element in our lives, yet we have so little serious consideration of breathing. You don't have to believe in Buddhism; you don't have to believe in anything. If you are Christian, then breathe Christ into you. You feel peace; you breathe out with compassion, with love. I think that this is essential. For those who can take time to breathe, then I would also say to make time to meditate, in whatever spiritual tradition is right for you. In contemplation we can see the people who are suffering and can understand their suffering, can see that they are as important as we are. Then I think some seeds are planted, not only for them but for our own benefit, as this brings very meaningful change.

General Jack Kidd, U.S.A.F. (Ret.)

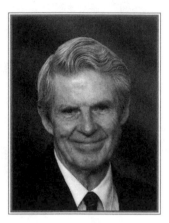

Following a distinguished career as a major general in the U.S. Air Force, General Kidd turned his attention to the United Nations and its role in peacekeeping throughout the world. In his contribution he shares his personal story and stresses the need for peace. "The plan proposed here has the potential for profound change in the world. The alternatives are clear."

A Change of Heart

As generals are known for giving the command to charge, to do battle, to win wars, it may seem odd that one was invited to contribute
to a book called *Voices from the Heart*. My thirty-one years in uniform
covered most all the bases: starting, fighting, operating, planning, and
ending wars, which in retrospect turned out to be an ideal exposure
for a very different agenda. My background included fighting in
World War II as a group operations officer and formation leader, on
one occasion leading General Curtis LeMay's entire force of about
240 bombers while less than four years out of college. During those
four years I instructed forty students in advanced flying training, became a squadron commander with twelve bombers and 350 men under my command, and flew lead formations of bombers all over
Europe. After the Berlin Airlift, I moved to join the Air Staff at the
Pentagon, recommending to the chief his positions on national war
plans—including those for World War III—or for his meetings with
the Joint Chiefs of Staff. I headed that office for four years. Then I
was with the Pacific Division of the Pentagon, implementing the
containment policy in the Pacific Ocean area, including helping
Vietnam against the Communist onslaught.

The day arrived when the Joint Chiefs of Staff were to decide whether to recommend deploying U.S. combat forces to Vietnam. I walked out of the Joint Staff office to go to the Air Staff to urge them to vote no. I was convinced that ground troops would become mired in the jungle terrain and this would severely limit effectiveness. Despite my convictions, once the decision was made, as head of office I wrote the message that started the movement of over 500,000 troops into Vietnam. I spent three years directing operations in Vietnam and throughout the Pacific area.

It was in retirement in the late 1970s that I began to question our political-military policies and to see the bigger picture. It has been an evolutionary process ever since. While war planning in the 1950s, I did not have a second thought about the growing nuclear arsenal; after all, the U.S. Air Force had a virtual monopoly. But later, as the U.S.-Soviet arms race burgeoned, it became obvious to me that it was a lose-lose situation. Each was being strained economically, but, more important, civilization itself was being placed at risk of oblivion. Contributing to my state of mind that nuclear weapons were useless was an event from active duty. As deputy chief of staff operations of the Air Force (Nuclear) Weapons Center, I chose to fly through the cloud of a thermonuclear burst within minutes of detonation in order to collect particulate samples for scientific analysis. It was an awesome experience.

During the early 1980s a series of events led to a deep personal change that resulted in what could be called a spiritual awakening. This allowed me to see and experience a still bigger picture: the oneness and sacredness of all life. Rooted in that reality, I made a conscious resolve to convert my background and skills of war planning to peace planning. Soon after that resolve, in 1984, I developed a plan for strategic cooperation between the United States and the U.S.S.R., including the elimination of nuclear weapons and cooperation in space.

In 1987, at the height of the Cold War, I was one of a group of fifteen retired Soviet and American generals and admirals which met in both Washington and Moscow. We came to the complete agreement that "nuclear weapons cannot be used for any rational military or political purpose. Actions to reduce nuclear weapons must be accelerated with the object of eliminating them entirely." More recently, about one hundred retired generals and admirals (including the original fifteen) from many different nations have gone on record saying that nuclear weapons are a detriment and that no military commander can assure winning a nuclear battle. May this step hasten the elimination of all nuclear weapons.

However, though the Cold War is over, the insidious spirits of fear, greed, arrogance, and confrontation are still in existence. This century has been six times bloodier than the last; the United States has been in a major war every sixteen years. I am deeply concerned that more is needed to prevent the recurrence of another arms race or war. *Homo sapiens* have continually found different and more efficient ways to maim and kill their own, starting with the stone, the club, and the bow and arrow and moving to the gun, the tank, poison gas, biological weapons, and the A-bomb. Now a single thermonuclear weapon is capable of causing whole cities to disappear. The detonation of thousands of such weapons would cause civilization as we know it to simply vanish and leave pockets of mutilated, disfigured, poisoned, and starving survivors in the global fallout. If a species of bugs had such a penchant for killing its own, it would be studied carefully to determine the source of such sadism. Is this notion of destruction exaggerated? No. Can it happen? Yes, simply by a national leader uttering a word or pushing a button.

The United States first built the A-bomb, followed by the Soviet Union; the same applies to the thermonuclear bomb, intercontinental ballistic missile (ICBM), and missile defense. Now a new, more efficient weapon is working its way to the drawing board. There seems to be a tacit understanding by military planners that the next big war will be in space; thus a futuristic space-based directed energy weapon is conceived as being able to wipe out a nation's war-making capacity, not in months or weeks but in hours. One can assume that such devastation would not only destroy steel and concrete but also kill countless humans. Naturally, many nations would want the capacity to destroy such a weapon suspended over their territory. The result could well be another arms race, this time in space.

We spent upward of $60 billion on Star Wars, with little if anything to show for it. Our government system now works to build weapons; then, when an enemy responds, it decides to take steps to get rid of them through arms control. How much intelligence does it take to outlaw even the concepts of weapons of mass destruction—before they're built—let alone eliminate mass destruction weapons already in existence?

About 110,000,000 people have been killed in wars in this century. If we added to that all the wounded, those made homeless, the bereaved, and those suffering the effects of war, the number could well exceed three-quarters of a trillion people. The U.S. toll this century is 640,000 Americans in uniform killed. In Korea and Vietnam, 100,000 Americans in uniform were killed. Korea remains as divided as it was forty-four years ago, and we still post 37,000 troops there; in Vietnam we simply walked away.

The story is not all bad. At least we agreed to reduce nuclear weapons in the Strategic Arms Reduction Treaties (START I and II) and the Intermediate Nuclear Force (INF) Treaty. The Anti-Ballistic Missile (ABM) Treaty of 1972 placed stringent limits on missile defenses, and there is now a new chemical weapons treaty. The massive destruction and chaos caused in World War II are behind us. For the first time in memory the world is free of the Cold War and ruthless, aggressive world powers. But more is necessary.

What is needed is a better amalgamation of defense, foreign policy, and arms reduction. We need a joint Defense/State/Arms Control and Disarmament Agency (ACDA) to thrash out issues together, rather than continue to highlight Defense as the prime agency for national security. If the joint Defense/State/ACDA spent one-hundredth, or even one-thousandth, of the current Defense Department's budget on preventive measures and arms reduction, it could create a national, long-range peace plan to eliminate weapons of mass destruction, promote an organization for verification of agreed arms reductions reporting to the U.N. Security Council, and develop with other nations a system for preventing the use of terrorist weapons. In other words, it is time to wage peace with all the vigor, zeal, and dedication with which wars have been waged for millennia.

The veto power of the five permanent members of the U.N. Security Council (China, Britain, France, Russia, and the United States) heads the list of things that must be changed. As no single nation should have the right to prevent the Security Council from carrying out its primary duty to maintain peace, any member of the council seen by the council to be in the act of committing or supporting aggression or posing a threat to peace should refrain from voting on a related issue. What is needed is a binding obligation that where there is a clear conflict of interest, the nation concerned will either excuse itself or be so required.

The Security Council has available several ways for effecting military action to deal with rogues. For instance, it can authorize the execution of an already unilaterally planned military operation or designate a nation to create a multilateral plan for dealing with a rogue nation. It can include safeguards to comply with nations' constitutional authority to declare war. The issues of command and control arrangements are rightfully sensitive and have been a major sticking point of any peace plan. Security Council planning should provide a political council of all involved nations to carry out its resolutions.

With the history of this century fresh in mind, all nations having the capacity to make nuclear and mass destruction weapons should welcome the opportunity to shed the burden of building these weapons while at the same time increasing their security, provided that there is satisfactory inspection and verification. An expanded and restructured U.N. International Atomic Energy Agency would be an appropriate body to take on the verification job.

Sovereignty is an issue as many nations fear the loss of freedom of action. However, the United States has entered into numerous treaties and pacts, all of which limit its sovereignty in some way. For example, under the two START pacts between the United States and Russia, nuclear weapons are being reduced mutually, so capability is being limited. The key point is that the decisions were made because both sides preferred reduction to the alternative.

The plan proposed here has the potential for profound change in the world. The alternatives are clear. If we do not proceed, the mistakes of history will be repeated. My friend and severest critic, a retired New York lawyer, says simply, "It won't work." My response to him is, "Neither of us knows whether it will work or how well it will work, but we must try."

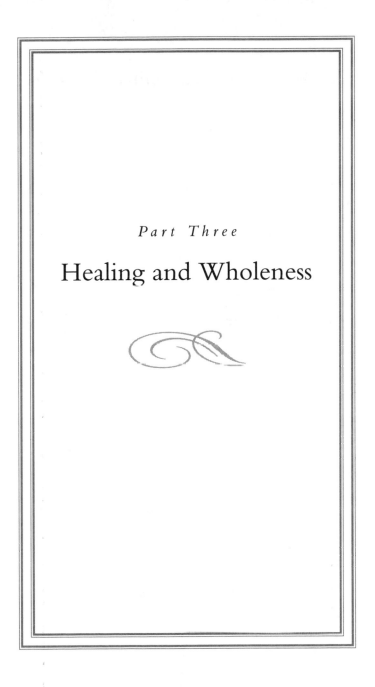

Part Three

Healing and Wholeness

Rachel Naomi Remen, M.D.

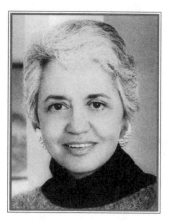

A lifetime of involvement with the medical world as both a doctor and patient has created in Rachel Naomi Remen a deep understanding of the healing process. In this piece she explores the vital role of spirit in healing. "After twenty years of working with people with cancer, watching them heal in a great variety of circumstances," she says, "I have come to suspect that healing is more closely related to mystery than mastery, more a function of the soul than of the mind."

Spirit

Resource for Healing

The field of mind-body health is almost twenty years old, and perhaps it is now time to admit that there are some serious limitations in thinking of the field in this way. After years of doing this work, I find that I am not at all certain that it is the mind that effects healing in many cases. Perhaps we might say that the mind is the highest human function but there is something in us that transcends our humanness and is the source of our healing. In speaking of mind-body health, we may risk overlooking this, or even forgetting it.

The term *mind-body health* suggests that healing occurs when we are able to use the mind to fix the body. Mobilizing the power of the mind seems to offer an attractive alternative to the intervention of the experts. To many it seems an easier, less painful, cheaper, and more efficient way to fix the body than surgery or other medical approaches. In a mastery-oriented culture, it also seems to offer the hope of greater personal control. Yet is healing a question of personal control, or may it be more a question of personal surrender? After twenty years of working with people with cancer, watching them heal in a great variety of circumstances, I have come to suspect that healing is more closely related to mystery than mastery, more a function of the soul than of the mind.

In pursuit of greater understanding of how we live, how consciousness and the body interact, the mechanism by which emotion affects the T-cells, or how the brain waves change when we pray, something very important may slip through our fingers, and we may not even know it. How we heal may be quite different from why we heal. Health is not an end; it is a means. Health enables us to serve our purpose in life, but it is not the purpose of life. Perhaps reconnecting to the purpose that we each serve may be the most powerful way to heal.

The real questions of health may not be questions of mechanism but questions of spirit. Healing is not a matter of mechanism; it is a work of spirit. At the very heart of spirit is mystery. Mystery is larger than the mind; it challenges the mind's dominion. Mystery is witnessed but never understood. The mind does not tolerate mystery with grace.

What happens when we base a healing system on an aspect of ourselves that cannot tolerate mystery? Contemporary allopathic medicine is the most intellectually oriented and analytical of the many healing systems we have developed in our pursuit of a response to suffering. It is the only healing system that does not allow for Divine intervention, the possibility of the mysterious or the miraculous. But the unexplained is a part of ordinary life. How does contemporary medicine respond when confronted with the unknown, the inexplicable, such as when someone recovers from an illness after all known means of cure have been exhausted?

Many years ago, when I was an intern, a man with widespread metastatic cancer was brought into our hospital to die. In those days before hospice he was admitted because he could not be cared for at home. I do not remember his name but I certainly remember his X rays. His bones were riddled with cancer, and there were great snowballs of tumor in both his lungs. In the two weeks he was in the hospital, all these cancer lesions disappeared and never came back.

Were we in awe? Certainly not. We were, if anything, frustrated. I remember the chief resident saying that we had most likely misdiagnosed this man, that he had not really had cancer. His biopsy slides were sent around the country to expert oncological pathologists. One by one they confirmed the original diagnosis. So we physicians gathered together in grand rounds to discuss this case. At this meeting of 250 physicians, it was concluded that the chemotherapy which had been completed a year before had suddenly worked. It would be ten years before I would remember this man's story and question this conclusion. Too great a rational objectivity can make you blind.

The mind has its limitations. When we are mentally identified, we have a tendency to deny that which cannot be understood. But much of what can be experienced and known can never be under stood. In valuing the rational as much as we do, we suffer from a culture-wide tendency to reject mystery, to ignore the spiritual dimensions of life, or to delegate spirit to others who we believe are better equipped to deal with it. But spirit cannot be delegated. We all participate in it. It is our deepest nature. There is no situation that is not a spiritual situation, no decision that is not a spiritual decision, no relationship that does not have a spiritual basis. All life is sacred. Life itself may serve some unknown purpose in which we all participate, knowing or unknowing.

Some of the people who have had a near-death experience report having found a greater sense of life's purpose. According to the near-death-experience literature, the purpose of life is deceptively simple. It is to grow in wisdom and to learn how to love better. We each have the opportunity to do this or not to do it. We may find the way to do it as a doctor, parent, clerk, bus driver . . . or not find it as a doctor, parent, clerk, bus driver. . . . And, of course, we may serve this purpose whether sick or well. If life serves this purpose, then health serves this purpose and illness can serve it also. We are offered a complete freedom of choice.

The mind is a fixer and deals in solutions. But healing is more an outcome of growth than an outcome of repair. Life is process. Broken is only a stage in that natural process. Fixing is a strategy appropriate only for the inanimate. When we fix people, we deny the power of the life in them and assert instead the power of our own expertise and our own skills. Fixing is a reductionist approach to life and certainly to suffering. Things that can never be fixed can still heal. We can grow beyond our suffering and often do. The following is the story of the first patient who taught me this.

Jed was a young man with osteogenic sarcoma of the right leg. He had been a high school and college athlete, and until the time of his diagnosis, his life had been good—beautiful women, fast cars, personal recognition. Two weeks after his diagnosis, they had removed his right leg above the knee. This surgery, which saved his life, also ended his life. Playing ball was a thing of the past.

He was a powerfully built and handsome young man, profoundly self-oriented and alienated. After his surgery, he had quit school and begun to drink heavily. When he first came to see me, he was filled with anger. He blamed everyone. Filled with a sense of injustice and self-pity, he hated all well people. In our second meeting, hoping to encourage him to talk more about himself, I gave him a pad and asked him to draw a picture of his body. He drew a crude sketch of a vase, just an outline. Running through the center of it, he drew a deep crack. He went over and over the crack with a black crayon, gritting his teeth and tearing the paper. He had tears in his eyes. They were tears of rage. It seemed to me that the drawing was a powerful statement of the pain and the finality of his loss. It was clear that this broken vase could never hold water, could never function as a vase again. It hurt to watch him. After he left, I folded the picture up and saved it; it seemed too important to throw away.

In time, his anger began to change in subtle ways. He began one session by handing me an item torn from our local newspaper. It was an article about a motorcycle accident in which a young man had lost his leg. His doctors were quoted at length. I finished reading and looked up. "Those idiots don't know the first thing about it," he said furiously. Over the next month he brought in more such articles. His reaction was always the same, a harsh judgment of the well-meaning efforts of doctors and parents. His anger about these other young people began to occupy more and more of our session time. No one understood them, no one was there for them, no one really knew how to help them. He was still enraged, but it seemed to me that underneath his anger a concern for others was growing. Encouraged, I asked him if he wanted to do anything about it. Caught by surprise, at first he said no. But later he asked me if I thought he could meet some of the others. I said that I would look into it. Within a few weeks, he began to visit young people in our hospital's surgical wards whose problems were similar to his own.

He came back from these visits full of stories, delighted to find he was able to reach others and be of help when no one else could. After a while he felt able to speak to parents and families and help them to understand better and to know what was needed. The surgeons, delighted with the results of these visits, referred more and more people to him. Some of these doctors had seen him play ball, and they began to spend a little time with him. As he got to know them, his respect for them grew. Gradually his anger faded and he developed a sort of ministry. I just watched and listened and appreciated him.

My favorite of all his stories concerned a visit to a young woman who had a tragic family history: breast cancer had claimed the lives of her mother, her sister, and her cousin. Another sister was in chemotherapy. This last event had driven her into action. At twenty-one she had both her breasts surgically removed.

He visited her in the hospital on a hot midsummer day wearing shorts, his artificial leg in full view. Deeply depressed, she lay in bed with her eyes closed. A radio on her bedside table was playing rock music. Everything he tried failed to reach her. She refused even to look at him. Frustrated, he finally stood, and in a last effort to get her attention he unstrapped his artificial leg and let it drop to the floor with a loud bang. Startled, she opened her eyes and saw him for the first time. Encouraged, he began to hop around the room, snapping his fingers in time to the music and laughing. She burst out laughing too. "Fella," she said, "if you can dance, maybe I can sing."

This young woman became his friend and began to visit people in the hospital with him. She was in school, and she encouraged him to return to school to study psychology and dream of carrying his work further. Eventually she became his wife, a very different sort of person from the models and cheerleaders he had dated in the past. But long before this we ended our sessions together. In our final meeting, we were reviewing the way he had come, the sticking points and the turning points. I opened his chart and found the picture of the broken vase he had drawn two years before. Unfolding it, I asked him if he remembered the drawing he had made of his body. He took it in his hands and looked at it for some time. "You know," he said, "it's not finished yet." Surprised, I extended my basket of crayons toward him. Taking a yellow crayon, he began to draw lines radiating from the crack in the vase to the very edges of the paper. Thick yellow lines. I watched, puzzled. He was smiling. Finally he put his finger on the crack, looked at me, and said softly, "This is where the light comes through."

Suffering often draws the soul close to us and enables us to find a greater wholeness in the midst of overwhelming loss. The power in suffering to promote integrity is not only a Christian belief; it is a part of almost every religious tradition. Yet, twenty years of working with people with cancer in the setting of unimaginable loss and pain suggests that this may not be a spiritual teaching or a religious belief at all, but rather some sort of natural law. That is, we might learn it not by Divine revelation but simply by a careful and patient observation of the world. Suffering shapes the life force, sometimes into anger, sometimes into blame and self-pity. Eventually it may show us the freedom of loving and serving life.

Indeed, denying spirit may be hazardous to your health. Much illness is attributed to stress, but perhaps the greatest source of stress is not overwork or unreasonable expectations. What we call stress may be a kind of spiritual isolation. Illness seems to uncover unrecognized spiritual needs, issues of alienation and depression, feelings people have that no one matters to them or that they matter to no one. In the setting of illness people may discover for the first time that a busy life has really been empty and that cherished goals have no real meaning. People may discover for the first time what is of real importance and live more courageously and fully.

The connection to the soul is often made through the heart. Spiritual isolation is living with a closed heart. It is epidemic in our culture. It has been surprising to observe how often the process of physical healing runs concurrent with the healing of the heart. A greater kindness, a greater compassion, seems to come naturally to many people as they work through severe illness.

Yitzak was a survivor. Liberated from a concentration camp in 1945, he had come to the United States, worked and studied hard, and was now a respected research chemist. Two years before, he had been diagnosed with cancer. Now he had come to Commonweal, our retreat for people with cancer, to see if he could engage and possibly defeat this enemy with the power of his mind, the aspect of his being that he trusted most profoundly.

At Commonweal we touch people and hug them a great deal more than was Yitzak's custom. Disconcerted at first, he would ask, "Vat is dis, all dis huggy-huggy? Vat is dis luff the strangers? Vat IS this?" But he let us hug him anyway. After a few days he began to hug us back.

The retreats last a week. By the fourth day the inner silence which has been slowly generated by daily Yoga practice has become very deep, and spontaneous insights often arise. Sometimes this silence allows people to find their healing for the first time. In the meditation which began the fourth morning session, Yitzak had an experience. It seemed to him that through his closed eyelids he could see a deep pinkish light, very beautiful and tender. Startled, he realized this light surrounded him and was coming in some mysterious fashion from his chest. The light had a direction; it was pouring out of his heart "like a big hemorrhage." He could not stop it, and when he realized this, he became frightened.

Yitzak had survived the concentration camps. A refugee, for many years he had lived, as it were, in a world of strangers. Since his experience as a boy, he had been very cautious with respect to his heart and loved only close people, only family. This way of living had helped him feel safer, had worked for him until now. But there is much fear behind such a wary lifestyle, and for the first time he had begun to feel this. It was not a comfortable feeling.

The staff dealt with his fear in the way we deal with everything else; we did not try to fix it, to explain away his experience, or to interpret it for him. Instead, we listened with interest and continued to support him as he tried to work out its meaning for himself. Over the next few days he seemed to relax more, to become more open.

Sunday, in the last meeting of the retreat, I try to tie up the loose ends. I knew Yitzak had been troubled by his experience, so I asked him how things were. He laughed. "Better," he said, and began to tell us of a walk he had taken on the beach the day before. In his mind, he had talked to God, asking God what all this was about, and had received comfort. Touched, I asked him what God had to say. He laughed again. "Ah, Rachel-le, I say to Him, 'God, is it OK to luff strangers?' And God says, 'Yitzak, vot is dis strangers? You make strangers; I don't make strangers.'"

Yitzak has established a generous scholarship so that anyone who wishes can attend the retreat. When asked if he wanted to choose those who received the money or to have them know his name, he said, "No. Just tell them it is from someone who cares about them, a friend."

There is no statute of limitations on healing. Forty years ago as a boy, Yitzak had closed his heart. Now, as he sought a healing for his body, he had begun to heal in other ways as well. In the acute struggle to survive our wounds, we may adapt a strategy of living that gets us through. But what we have done to survive may be quite different than what we need to do in order to live fully. Life-threatening illness may cause us to reexamine the very premises on which we have based our lives, perhaps freeing ourselves from those premises for the first time.

The process of illness, limitation, and suffering, the shocking isolation of a brutal disease may awaken in us the seeker, who is so much more than the scientist. We begin to sort values, leaving behind those which have been outgrown, which do not support life. People who have never considered such things before find themselves reaching for a sense of personal meaning in their pain, intuitively aware that in times of crisis meaning is strength. Ultimately they may come to know of the uniqueness and value of their own lives, the uniqueness and value of every life. That value is often rooted in a sense of mystery.

A human being is not a mechanism, but an opportunity for the Infinite to manifest. The mind's need for mastery can stifle our sense of mystery, can blind us to the mystery around us, and in doing so, alienate us from the true direction of our healing. A week after a sixteen year-old girl died of leukemia, her mother brought me the following poem in a sealed envelope. She had left it for me in her will.

Cancer.
I disappear,
devoured by the pain.
I know
I am a speck,
a mote of dust dancing in a sunbeam.
I know my little dance matters.
My life
serves Life
Itself.

Dean Ornish, M.D.

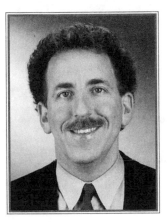

ollowing his own early experience with depression, Dean Ornish realized that suffering was a powerful doorway to personal transformation. In this moving article he shares his insights into illness and healing. "For me the epidemic in our culture is not only physical heart disease but also emotional and spiritual heart disease," he states. "This is where the suffering is the deepest and the healing the most profound."

Doorways for Transformation

During my first year of premedical college, I experienced great suffering, despair, and emotional depression. In that environment people tend to define their self-esteem and net worth by how well they perform academically. One of the things that the school catalogue didn't tell us was that the school had the highest per capita suicide rate of any school in the country.

Our organic chemistry professor taught without any conceptual basis to his teaching. He started out on the first day of class telling us, "This is a weed-out course, and I'm going to weed you out," and proceeded to do just that. I can think conceptually but I don't memorize that well, and we were being given one unrelated chemistry equation after another to remember. Since this was the most important course in determining whether one would be accepted in medical school, I began to worry that I wasn't doing well enough, and the more I worried the harder it was to study. It became a vicious cycle. I began to get extremely agitated to the point where I was having a hard time sleeping. It got worse and worse until I ended up not sleeping for a week straight and got so agitated and confused that I wasn't able to read a headline on a newspaper, much less memorize a number of chemistry equations.

I began to feel like I was going to fail, that I wasn't going to get accepted into medical school and so I was never going to amount to anything. But worse than this crisis of confidence was a spiritual vision that I had at that time. It was that nothing was going to bring me lasting happiness. I had been taught by my culture and my family that if I became a doctor and I married a beautiful woman and I became rich and famous, then these things would bring lasting happiness, and yet I knew that they wouldn't. That was a bad combination: feeling that I wasn't going to amount to anything and that even if I did, it wouldn't matter anyway. It left me profoundly depressed.

I remember sitting in class one day and saying to myself, "I know what. I'll just kill myself; that will take care of it all." It felt like a wonderful release; that something as extreme as committing suicide might bring me the peace that I was so sorely lacking. I began making plans and first thought I could jump off the oil derrick that was in front of the rather sterile apartment complex in which I lived. But I realized that would make a big mess and everybody would know I had committed suicide and my parents would be upset. So I thought I would get drunk and then drive at a hundred miles an hour into the side of a bridge, and everybody would think I was just a drunk driver. But having run myself down so badly, I actually got a case of infectious mononucleosis, so I didn't even have the energy to kill myself. Eventually I withdrew from school and went home.

The plan was to go to Dallas and recuperate until I was strong enough to go out and kill myself, as crazy as that sounds. Meanwhile my older sister had been training with an Indian yogi and eminent spiritual teacher, Swami Satchidananda. My parents had noticed the improvement in her life, so when Swamiji came to Dallas, they decided to have a cocktail party for him. This was unusual back then, in 1972, especially in Dallas. He walked into our living room and said, "Nothing can bring you lasting happiness," which of course I had already figured out, except that he looked pretty happy and I looked miserable. He went on to say what is by now a New Age cliché but at that time turned my life around, which is that "nothing can bring you lasting happiness, but you have that already if you just stop disturbing it." He went on to say how in the process of running after those things that you think will make you happy, which was, in my case, getting into medical school, you end up disturbing what you have already. It is one of life's supreme ironies, like the musk deer that wanders through the forest looking for the source of the scent it can smell without realizing that it comes from itself.

I figured that this was worth a try and I could always kill myself if it didn't work, so I began practicing Yoga and meditation. I started getting little glimpses of what it felt like to be more at ease and see-ing that it came not from getting something that I thought I needed but rather from quieting down my mind enough to stop disturbing it. And once I made that connection, realizing that it wasn't some-thing that I got but something that I already had, I stopped asking, "What can I get to make me happy?" and started asking, "What am I doing that is disturbing my peace and well-being?"

For me this made all the difference in the world. I went back to school and graduated first in my class; I changed my major from bio-chemistry to humanities and ended up giving the commencement address. I say this simply to illustrate having experienced both ex-tremes of the spectrum, from when I thought that I had to do well to get into medical school so that I could be a doctor in order to feel good about myself and be able to say, "Hey, look at me, I'm worthy of your love and respect" but being so distressed that I couldn't even memorize a newspaper headline, to when I began to get just little glimpses of peace and joy and well-being and was able to think clearly enough to be able to perform at a very high level.

I went to medical school and studied bypass surgery. At first it was exciting and dramatic, but over time it became a metaphor of an in-complete approach, that we were literally bypassing the problem without dealing with the underlying causes. People would come in, we would operate on them, and their chest pains would get better. But then they would go off and smoke and eat the same foods and get stressed and not exercise, and more often than not their bypasses would clog up again. I knew it wasn't because the surgeon wasn't good but because there was something inherently limited in the process itself. We were bypassing the problem, a little like mopping up the floor around a sink that's overflowing without first turning off the faucet.

That metaphor has continued throughout my work. Sometimes we do need to mop up the floor—drugs and surgery can be lifesaving in a crisis, but they are only temporary; they do not address the cause. If we do not address the underlying cause, then more often than not the same problem comes back again or we get a new set of problems or side effects we hadn't counted on. We may be faced with painful choices. Up to half the bypass grafts clog up again within three to five years, and up to 50 percent of the angioplastied arteries clog up again within four to six months. We now spend eighteen to twenty billion dollars a year in the United States on bypass surgery.

The most meaningful part of my work has been not just to show scientifically that the progression of heart disease can often be stopped or reversed by making changes in diet and lifestyle through Yoga and meditation, moderate exercise, psychosocial support, and a low-fat vegetarian diet. These are important, but what I find most personally gratifying are those aspects that are more difficult to measure. People may come into our program because they want to unclog their arteries, lose weight, get their blood pressure down, lower their cholesterol, reduce their need for insulin, and so on, but what sustains them is that they begin to rediscover inner sources of peace and joy and well-being. Although that's more difficult to measure than cholesterol or blood pressure, it's probably the most meaningful for the patients.

So, having survived being profoundly depressed during college, what this experience taught me is that suffering, whether emotional, physical, or both, can be a doorway for transforming our lives in ways that go beyond just the physical, beyond what even we thought we wanted. For me it was profound depression; for someone else it might be heart disease or cancer, although in most cases the physical suffering is just the tip of the iceberg. The reason why suffering can be a doorway for transformation is if you are in enough pain and if the strategies for numbing or killing or distracting yourself from that pain are no longer working, then the idea of change becomes more attractive and the status quo is no longer so acceptable. The beauty is that most people find they feel better, not only physically. They get glimpses of what it means to be more at peace, and they realize that it comes not from something that they thought they needed but rather from ceasing to disturb what they have already.

For me the epidemic in our culture is not only physical heart disease but also emotional and spiritual heart disease. Think of how loneliness, isolation, and depression are so common, with the breakdown of the social networks that used to give us a sense of connection and community. This is where the suffering is the deepest and the healing the most profound. One woman in our study said, "I've got twenty friends in a packet of cigarettes and they're always there for me, and nobody else is. You're going to take away my twenty friends? What are you going to give me?" One man said, "I've got friends I go see at the bar every day. Jack Daniels, Jim Beam, Johnny Walker, they're always there for me." It's no accident that beer commercials always have people drinking in a group of friends. No one sits in a bar and drinks by her- or himself in a commercial.

In our culture suffering is viewed as the enemy to be killed. When I was training, if somebody came into the emergency room and was in the middle of having chest pains or a heart attack, we were told to kill the pain as quickly as possible, without first listening to the pain, which is like killing the messenger that brings bad news without hearing what the message is. My experience is that suffering is information. If we listen to it, if we pay attention to it, there is so much we can learn from it. And if we listen to the milder forms of suffering, then we can often avoid the more profound ones later. It is like a ship that has drifted a little off course. If we notice when it is drifting just a little, then it doesn't take much to get it back on course; if we don't pay attention, then the ship can drift thousands of miles out to sea.

I believe that the universe provides us with opportunities to learn and to grow in wisdom and compassion. It is as if the universe is saying, "Hey! Wake up! Pay attention! There is something that you're doing that is not in your best interests." And if we don't take any notice, then those messages get louder and the pain gets more profound, whether it is physical, emotional, spiritual, or all three. Suffering is not a punishment; it is simply information that we can use to make a judgment. We have so many ways of trying to kill the pain, to distract ourselves or numb the pain, whether through cigarettes, alcohol, or other drugs, by eating too much, working too hard, or even channel surfing. We have many ways to escape temporarily from the pain, but it is always temporary. So the pain comes back even stronger because we haven't dealt with the reason for it.

One of the obstacles that we had when we were doing research on this was raising funds to do it, not only because people thought it was impossible to reverse heart disease but because they thought it was equally impossible that people would change their diet and lifestyle. They'd say, "We can't even get our patients to eat less red meat. You're expecting them to be vegetarian, to do Yoga and meditation, and to quit smoking all at the same time? There's no way people can do that."

But we work at deeper levels. We don't just say, "Do this, do that, don't do this, don't do that," because we have learned that even more than being healthy, people want to feel free and in control. As soon as I tell somebody not to do something, he or she immediately wants to do it. It's just human nature. It goes all the way back to Adam and Eve. The very first dietary intervention failed when God said, "Don't eat the apple." I can't do better than God, so I don't try. What I do say is, "Look, you're an adult; whatever you want to do is fine. It's your life and you're the one who has to take the consequences for it and I will support whatever you choose." They are more likely to make changes if I don't insist on their making them, because then they are making them for themselves, not for me. If they see that I have an investment in getting these changes, they're going to fight me, and they will feel like they are disappointing me if they don't make the changes that I feel they ought to be making.

By working on the emotional, psychosocial, behavioral, and spiritual dimensions, it becomes easier for people to make changes because they reframe the reason for making them. It's not just about risk-factor reduction or about living for a few months longer, it's about making changes that enhance the quality of life. They discover inner sources of peace, joy, and well-being, a sense of connection and unity with people. We have support groups so people can talk about how they're feeling without fear that somebody is going to judge, criticize, reject, or abandon them, and that is all about enhancing a sense of intimacy and ending the isolation. If somebody feels like the only friends that he or she has are the twenty in a packet of cigarettes, it can be very hard to get that person interested in quitting smoking. But if we create structures that provide people with a sense of supportive community, as well as techniques to help them quiet down their mind and body, then we find that they are letting go of something that they don't need any more as opposed to engaging in a daily battle of struggle, self-denial, and deprivation.

A year ago I was running in the Bay-to-Breakers race in San Francisco. It's a seven-and-a-half-mile race with forty thousand people in it. At about the six-mile point I saw a man collapse in the street from a heart attack. I started doing some CPR, another doctor that I knew also stopped, a paramedic brought a defibrillator, and we shocked the heart, got it started again, put him on an IV and gave him some drugs, and sent him off for an emergency bypass operation. I didn't feed him vegetables or teach him meditation, because what he needed was a defibrillator, drugs, and surgery to save his life. But to me that is the beginning, not the end. Later he came and spent a week with us at our residential program so he could learn how to take care of himself and improve his whole life.

The techniques we use—stretching, breathing, meditation, Yoga, and a low-fat vegetarian diet—were not developed by the ancient swamis and rabbis, the priests, monks, and nuns in order to lower their cholesterol or blood pressure or so they could perform better in the boardroom, although they can help us do all those things. Rather, they are really powerful tools for transformation, giving us the direct experience, even if only temporarily, of what it means to feel more at ease and more at peace.

Healing is something that occurs in the spirit, a healing of the isolation that separates us from each other and our nature. We can make our world either a heaven or a hell; those who see the spirit in themselves and each other make the world a heaven. They discover how suffering can be a doorway for transforming their lives in ways that ultimately can make them not only healthier but also more meaningful. Much of the effort that we make as physicians or health professionals is based on lengthening life, but we first need to ask more important questions such as: Why do we want to live longer? What is our purpose in life? What is the meaning? Why are we here? These are the questions that I wrestled with when I was younger. While the answers remain a mystery, the search for answers has opened doors in my life that have enabled me to feel more truly alive.

Sheila Cassidy, M.D.

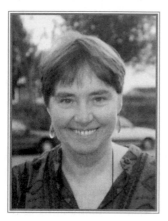

Sheila Cassidy is particularly familiar with pain, having been tortured in Chile for helping a wounded soldier. Here she shares her personal story and her experiential sense of what is needed by those who are suffering. "A great deal of accompanying people with pain," she states, "is about finding the person who has been half-destroyed and communicating with her or him."

Accompanying People in Pain

In 1972 I went to South America on a cargo boat in order to work in a hospital in Chile and found myself caught in the middle of the military coup. I treated a man who was on the run and as a result I ended up in prison. During the course of one night I was tortured repeatedly with electric shocks while I was naked, blindfolded, and spread-eagled on a metal bunk. One electrode was placed in my vagina and another, a pincer, used randomly across my body. This went on for many hours in their attempt to get information from me. Then they put me in solitary confinement for three weeks followed by five weeks in a detention camp. I spent much of this time in prayer, presenting God with my anguish and fear for both myself and my fellow prisoners. The presence of God was very real to me during those hard weeks, and the conviction that God is with us always and everywhere has remained with me to this day.

When I came back, I spent a long time doing human rights lecturing and then decided to try my vocation as a nun. But I found it extremely difficult living in a community entirely of women, and eventually they threw me out because I was so miserable. Then I tried to be a hermit on my brother's farm, but after a little while I ran out of money, and, as the only thing I knew how to do was to be a doctor, I went back to medicine. To my great amusement, I found that was where I belonged, not in a convent or a hermitage but in a hospital.

Eventually I became the medical director of the new Plymouth Hospice for people with advanced cancer. We started off with seven beds in a private house and slowly enlarged it to a twenty-bed, purpose-built hospice. Now I'm doing psychosocial oncology, which is providing emotional and psychological support for cancer patients.

Because of what happened to me in Chile, I have no fear of being alongside people in pain. I feel drawn to them in the same way that other people feel repelled, because I can see the real person underneath. I am with the person, not the pain. The dignity of each human being is intrinsic: either we can acknowledge it in the way we treat people or we can completely ignore it. But we can't remove people's dignity from them. I was stripped naked and tortured and ended up kneeling down begging for mercy. I felt extremely stupid, but I did not lose my dignity through being broken or violated. In respecting people—acknowledging their human dignity—we are recognizing the Divine within them.

It is important to have some idea of the impact of illness on people's lives: getting cancer, or AIDS, or motor neurone disease is like having a bomb drop on your life. Working with such patients is like working in the rubble caused by the bomb. If you look very carefully under rubble, sometimes you find people still alive. In the same way we have to look under the neurotic, angry, desperate person for that personality which has been bombed in under the pain. A great deal of accompanying people with pain is about finding the person who has been half-destroyed and communicating with her or him. My uncle was a highly intelligent, dignified man. When he had a stroke, it was very hard to see underneath the pathetic and confused man sitting in a room full of old people. It's so easy to lose sight of the person inside.

When people develop a life-threatening disease, such as cancer, they come slap up against their own mortality. Aleksandr Solzhenitsyn talks about the moment of arrest, of being catapulted into another existence. Suddenly you realize you may not live forever. It brings up so many philosophical and emotional questions that may never have been considered before. But more than anything, it produces an absolute terror and a very deep sense of loss.

It is like a journey into the unknown. You don't know what is going to happen. You don't know if you're going to die, you don't know what the treatment is going to be like, you don't know if you're going to hold up emotionally. So people need accompanying. I like to have what I call a covenant relationship, particularly with the terminally ill, because they are very vulnerable to emotional distress. A covenant relationship in the Old Testament, scriptural sense is what God has with his people. Accompanying people with cancer, particularly the dying, and the bereaved, is almost like a marriage. It's for better, for worse, for richer, for poorer.

We show respect for people by trying to find and then meet their needs. We all have primitive physiological needs: for food, rest, shelter, relief from pain, going to the toilet—all that very basic human stuff. We ignore these basic needs at our peril. If we don't attend to them, we can't deal with the higher, more creative social and spiritual needs.

The most primitive fear of the human being is to be abandoned, so people need to know that there is someone there for them. This need is particularly in evidence when people are very sick. It is the need to belong, to have someone to confide in, the need for someone whom they can depend on, whom they can trust. And these needs are made much more pressing by illness. There's something very powerful about a relationship of attunement that makes people feel good, makes them feel safe and heard. In the same way that a mother provides an attachment figure of security for the child, so if we have someone to whom we can be attached in adult life, then we are better able to face the difficult times.

Sometimes partners can't cope; sometimes they are too distressed themselves to listen. It doesn't always work that the person you love most can support you. So you can imagine that there is a loss of that security alongside a sense of vulnerability, a loss of well-being, of good looks, of job, even of continence. It is a whole experience of loss. The person who accompanies the patient is, as it were, walking with them along this very narrow way, accompanying them through this very scary experience.

The anger goes very deep. Being able to cope with someone's anger is a fundamental thing in accompanying. There is a sense of powerlessness against the doctors. You come to see the doctor with a list of questions and you get so scared you can't ask them, or you get confused, or you didn't ask the one question you wanted to. There is also the sense of powerlessness against fate. Whether you see it as God or a sort of Divine force or nothing, there are always the endless questions: Why me? How can there be a God if this is happening to me? How can there be a loving God if my child is dying?

I have no problem reconciling the fact of pain with the existence of God because my concept of God is of a very wild, mysterious, transcendent god. The whole thing of the mystery of the creation and of suffering is infinitely bigger than we can understand, and I am very comfortable living with that mystery. For me, the Divine encompasses the transcendent and the immanent. And so God is the totally unknowable, mysterious Creator, but God is also "as near as the neck of my camel," as the Muslims say. God is within me, so when I suffer, God suffers. It is important to feel free to be angry with God; he is well able to cope with our fury.

I have an image of God as the wheelchair God, the powerless God. This is the mystery that we cannot get our minds around. The whole thing is a paradox; it doesn't make sense. But I have sufficient faith, sufficient experience of the Divine, to believe in it. For me everything is a manifestation of God, and the whole of life is a monumental revelation. If I see badness, I usually see it as very sick and wounded people. If you scratch the surface of the torturer or the child molester, you will find a wounded person underneath.

When a child is born, particularly when it is very young, the way it is held is very important. There is something equally important about the way we hold people when we treat them. If you are very frightened, what you want is either to disappear under your bed covers or to be held by your beloved. The covers are a poor substitute for having someone who will put his or her arms around you and say, "It'll be okay." Hugging people is being in a relationship with them, having a listening, attuned relationship. For frightened people the secure base is in being held.

The counseling relationship is the holding relationship par excellence; by listening and not being completely fazed or distressed ourselves, we are able to contain other people's distress. That relationship is what I call the "safe space," a relationship in which they can say whatever they like. They can say "I hate that doctor" or "I hate this illness" or "I wish my wife would cope better." They can say the unsayable and think the unthinkable and know that they will not be rejected. That relationship is one in which we walk fearlessly alongside people and help them at each stage of the journey, help them to accept their reality, by not lying, not giving false encouragement, false consolation, false reassurance. It includes not forcing things down their throats, but being there to comfort them as the truth dawns on them and answering their questions honestly. Most people cope much better if they know what is happening.

We must learn to listen with our eyes, our ears, and our hearts. Listening with the eyes is looking clearly and recognizing when people are utterly exhausted because they haven't slept for days, when they are vibrating with fear, when they are very sick, when they have stopped looking after themselves, seeing the signs of tension, depression, and unhappiness. For instance, a man in our clinic was obviously absolutely terrified, so I took him to one side and said, "You're very scared, aren't you?" He said yes. It turned out that when he was eight he was buried in the Blitz. He very nearly suffocated as they tried to dig him out, and he had to scrabble his way out with his bare hands. Now that he knew that he was dying, he had nightmares every night about being buried alive. He used to wake up with pains in his fingers. Once he was able to talk it through and we were able to give him some fairly heavy night sedation, he was able to sleep. But if I hadn't been so convinced that this man was absolutely scared, we would have missed it.

Listening with the ears is listening to the words chosen, the tone of the voice, the sort of hesitation when someone is talking about something he or she is ashamed of, the story line going through the words, the underlying theme and trying to pick up any anger or bitterness and pull it into the light, or any self-pity or guilt. It includes listening to the silences. The big mistake that we all make at the beginning of this kind of work is to talk too much. We have to learn how to listen to people and give them time to process what they are saying. Undivided attention is really about attunement. It's about putting aside our own difficulties and just being there for another. Accompanying people with cancer is trying to be a rock in the background, so that they know that there is someone there to support them if something terrible happens.

There's a sense in which people have every right to be afraid of death. Each person faces death in her or his own way, but I think that everybody who approaches it is scared until they come to some kind of adjustment. However, most people are utterly shattered, devastated, at whatever age, when they find out that they are going to die. We have a basic coping strategy, which is that death is something that happens to other people. We ignore death until it comes.

We need not be afraid of being normal with dying people or with bereaved people. It is a great lack in society that people are shunned because we don't know what to say to them. I am surrounded by death but also by life. Working with the dying is working with life, not death. It's living life as fully as is humanly possible until we die. Because the relationships I have with my patients are often quite short, we live them very fully.

We can listen to God in all sorts of different ways. When it comes down to the crunch, it's really all about love, isn't it? "Where true love is, God is dwelling." Love is like a basket of loaves and fishes; you never have enough until you start to give it away.

Stephen Levine

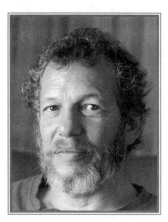

*S*tephen Levine has for more than twenty years offered counseling to the terminally ill and insights on healing through his many best-selling books. In his contribtution he shares the essence of healing. "Discovering the truth of pain, surrendering to pain, does not mean letting the pain eat us alive," he tells us. "It means softening around it, letting go of that which turns pain into suffering, letting go of the places where there is resistance."

A Vow of Responsibility to the Heart

I don't think that many people come to the spiritual path because they just swoon when they think of God. Most people come because they—we—need help. There is a tremendous amount of guilt and grief—unresolved grief—in those who come to the path. Life can be more painful than we can sometimes bear. We get stressed because we can't get what we want, so the very nature of desire becomes suffering. Desire is not good or bad, just painful. Good and bad is our unresolved grief, unresolved self-hatred, our shame and guilt. It's not that we are good or bad. Human beings are absolutely gorgeous when they are not stressed, and that's the proof that they are essentially good.

Frustration is the biggest of all stresses. On the one hand, frustration could say the old way just doesn't work anymore, and that is a wonderful, though very painful, realization. But usually frustration leads to aggression or fear. Very few people can stay indifferent to their states of mind. The very nature of wanting is the feeling of incompleteness, of helplessness, and to some degree of hopelessness. And then it flips over so that most of our hope becomes based on fear, and when we try to apply hope to illness, it usually makes it worse.

Normally, the first thing we do when pain arises is harden to it. We try to ostracize the part of our body or our mind that is in pain. The more we tighten against or resist pain, the more it turns into suffering. Pain is a given in life, while suffering is part of the momentum of our unresolved grief. Every time we are in pain, it stimulates grief. Discovering the truth of pain, surrendering to pain, does not mean letting the pain eat us alive. It means softening around it, letting go of that which turns pain into suffering, letting go of the places where there is resistance. When we withdraw our attention from pain, we never get insight into it, insight into the deeper level of connection with what caused that pain or can heal it. We can start to meet pain with mercy instead of hatred.

Watch pain settle as you soften and start to recondition your response to it. Watch what happens when you start to send mercy and loving-kindness into little pains. Let your heart start to connect with the pain, instead of letting your mind close around it. Let there be the possibility of real feelings, real healing. The healing we took birth for.

Anyone in a relationship is going to have frustration. When you get used to it, then you can say, "Big surprise, here's the old human stuff again." When you are relating to it instead of from it, there is really space for both of you to have your beliefs and your hearts. Don't try to resolve differences. As an experiment take three months in which you do not try to resolve your differences; rather, explore together the nature of difference, the nature of discord. Two people who disagree and keep their hearts open is a miracle in this world.

How do you open your heart? We start by learning to just breathe in and out of the heart, focusing on the breath in the heart, entering into that breath. I don't know how anybody stays alive without a practice of breathing, of being in the moment. My feeling is that love is the only rational act of a lifetime. And how we learn to be loving is by watching how angry we are. We see that the mind has a will of its own, and it doesn't always have our best interest at heart. It is driven by a desire for immediate satisfaction.

If we can deal with the five- and ten-pound weights—the smaller, lighter griefs or frustrations or angers—the more options we have for investigation. We can't approach a blazing fire; we'd just get burned to death. But we can approach a match. We can approach a flashlight. We can approach a small fire. So instead of suppressing the five- and ten-pound angers, instead of making out, "I'm a good person, I'm not angry," we get to know the anger. We open, soften to that anger. Let it float. Start to relate to it instead of from it. Watch, here comes frustration; there it is, yes, and there's anger. Start to relate to it from a merciful space, start to see yourself a little bit as God might see you, with great compassion.

You start to learn the nature of anger. You don't try to make it go away. It is time to stop abusing that pain. It is time to start treating that pain like it was our only child, to start embracing it. Yes, we wish it had never happened and we can go crazy wishing it had never happened, but the pain is there; the experiences are there. If you are involved with analyzing—how could this happen to me, and so on— you will never free yourself. You will never free the child who is abused; you will do very little to decrease the tendency toward abuse in the world.

If you start to see how much pain you are in and to meet your pain with mercy, then you will be free. There is no desire we have that is stronger than to protect the innocent and the weak, so of course the frustration is going to be rage, absolute rage, if they are abused or hurt. But you soften around it; it's okay that you are raging. Notice how it hardens with another thought, softening, hardening, ten thousand moments of losing it, ten thousand and one moments of letting go, letting it just be there—mercy for yourself; you are in pain. It's that simple, just you in pain. Now turn toward that other human being who is in pain and have mercy. Send mercy into their pain.

To say to someone whose child has been abused that he or she should forgive the abuser is insane and abusive if he or she has not yet softened to the anger. First we have to forgive ourselves for being so angry. Naturally we are angry; we are even angrier than we know we are. But we have mercy for ourselves; we do not have to hate. Fearlessness is the willingness to let fear be in the mind and the ability to enter it wholeheartedly. Fearlessness is not the necessity for fear to go away. Fearlessness is that fear doesn't stop us from opening, from softening. True fearlessness is love. Love is the absence of fear, when the heart is wide open.

When we acknowledge our suffering, we realize we are not crazy because we are suffering so much. Everybody is suffering. As you read these words, your mind says, yes, but nobody knows how much I'm suffering! Just watch how attached you are to your suffering, how identified you are with it. We refuse to let go of our suffering. The irony of the whole game is we say we only want to be happy, but letting go of our suffering is the hardest thing to do. It means letting go of our identity, our me-ness.

Try living the next year as though it were your last. You have just this one more year. We don't see much death in the real, in the flesh; we are not at ease with the reality of death. Our fear of death is more a fear of violence than it is of just dying in our sleep. We seldom have dreams of dying easily or painlessly; rather, we fantasize a car accident or another sudden, violent death. The more materialist a society is, the greater its fear of death. That has no relationship to the reality of death, to the flesh of death, to the smell of death, to the touch of death, to the extraordinary beauty and exquisite loving-kindness of some closures.

Where are we going? What is our direction? We have to watch our motivation for the next step. Why are we taking the next step? Is it pointing toward what brings us real joy or is it pointing toward only momentary pleasure? We have to investigate this addiction to momentary pleasure as one of the greatest causes of suffering. The whole concept of happiness based on fulfilling pleasure is really a superstition, for joy is our birthright and that has to be unconditional, not based on anything. Are you moving toward momentary happiness, momentary pleasure, or are you moving toward something that is essential joy? Joy is a deeper and deeper discovery of wider and wider levels of being that occur as we go beneath the level of ordinary awareness.

It's very important to know why we are doing something, to know our inner motivation, just to see it and name it as a state of mind. What is the state of mind in which that act is taken? In taking a step forward, one person takes that step in fear whereas another takes that step in love. Who do we think is going to be able to embrace the beloved? One whose heart is wide enough to embrace even that which is beyond her- or himself? Or one who is trying to control, is looking for happiness in a place too small to contain God? The more we see what causes our personal suffering, the greater our heart connection with others who are also suffering.

The pain of forty thousand children starving to death is on so many levels. The burning in the stomach that each child feels is the burning in the stomach I feel. On one level we can experience their pain. On another level we can see that it is greed that has kept those children's plates empty. What is greed based on? Ignorance. Ignorance is thinking you are the mind. Ignorance is thinking I am I and you are you. Ignorance is us and them. Ignorance is anything other than the nondual truth of essential reality. To the degree I am not in my essence, I am in such pain. We are all in such pain. What those children are experiencing is the aftermath of the attachment to ourselves: our fear that we are not going to get another meal, our fear that our grandchildren are not going to go to college. Our greed takes the last piece of bread off the table of those children.

Those people who are locking their grain silos are not bad. They are just afraid. When we are talking about dying, when we are talking about people getting along in relationship, when we are talking about how to work with physical pain, it always comes down to the same thing: our relationship to fear. If we want to open our hearts to dying, if we want to open our hearts to those forty thousand children who are starving, we have to have learned to keep our hearts open in hell. The only way to do that is to relate directly to fear instead of reacting unconsciously from fear.

This means becoming responsible for ourselves and our world. The word responsibility has caused so many problems. We've mixed responsibility with blame. My sense of responsibility is the ability to respond instead of the compulsion to react. When I can't do anything for a starving child, when I can't put food into that child's mouth, I can still bring that child into my heart in my prayers and in my meditation. This opens my heart, creating at least one less chance that I will act out of greed or selfishness. To be responsible is to try to stay soft, to respond to the situation. To be responsible means you can feel hopeless but you are never really helpless. You always have the alternative of softening, of opening your heart, of sending lovingkindness to somebody.

I was doing in-service at a hospice in Texas. They said they wanted me to see a woman who had been in a full coma for many days. They thought she would have died weeks ago but she hadn't. She was from the poor part of western Texas, with seven children under ten years old and an alcoholic husband. She had very advanced cancer. The nurses had been going to her and telling her it's okay to die. They were reacting to her condition, but they weren't responding to her. They went in with a menu, with an agenda; even though they were good words, they weren't appropriate in that moment.

I sit next to her on the bed. She's in pin-stick unresponsive coma, that heavy kind of almost snore-breathing coma. And I say to her that I know everybody has been telling her it's all right to die and I know she feels it's not all right to die. I say, "You've got seven children under ten years old and an alcoholic husband, and you cannot imagine for the life of you how this is going to work out after you die. It wasn't very good before, so how can it get better without you?" And I notice the breathing changing just a little bit. I continue to talk to her and I respond to her, entering into responsibility to this other human being. And I tell her, "I've seen it happen so many times before. I've seen many children with difficult fathers. And you will be amazed how the children will pull together." And I told her some stories about children pulling together and helping the father and maintaining the home. As I was talking to this woman in a full coma, tears are pouring out from under her closed eyelids.

I could have walked in there and said it's okay to die. But you have to go in there not knowing. To be responsible, you have to not know. She died within a couple of hours. With so many children, they will do what they have to do. A seven-year-old is a whole human being. And when you see so many children working together, the love is astounding.

We see the forests dwindling, violence increasing, trust diminishing, and we ponder what our responsibility might be in such a confused and confusing world. We have only the smallest idea of how to deal with the avalanche of problems that confronts us. We have forgotten or dismissed the source of our greatest power, our deepest clarity, our broadest compassion. We have forgotten our responsibility to our hearts.

Recognizing that responsibility is the ability to respond, we acknowledge that responsibility itself is more a quality of the healing heart than of the conflicted mind. And so we vow to take responsibility for the quality of responsibility, to embrace the qualities of the opening heart rather than the rusted machinations of the ever-defensive mind. Our world is a manifestation of our vows; a vow is the effort it takes to become effortless.

We take responsibility by softening the belly and taking a few breaths into the heart. We quiet down enough to hear the subtle whispers. We open to a storehouse of intuition to discover answers to questions of survival and sanity too big for the small mind. And so a second vow arises: to explore and release that in the mind which obstructs this deeper flow. It means letting go of our suffering. This is the hardest work we will ever do; it is the beginning of relieving the suffering of the world.

A vow to stay open is the salvation of the future. Such a vow acts as a platform from which to make the leap of faith into the heart, to practice kindness and forgiveness, to cultivate gratitude and merciful awareness, to keep the heart open in hell, to keep the heart open even to the moments it is closed. Thus the essential vow is that nothing, but nothing, is worth the heart's being closed for even a moment longer!

If we take responsibility now for our enormous hearts, all our questions will be answered in the moment of their arising. Our deepest wisdom, our unending connectedness with all that lives, will effortlessly present itself. It is a response in our hearts to the heart, a vow of personal responsibility to the universal, a commitment to the healing we took birth for.

We are not separate. There is no pain in someone else that is not somewhere in us. We are not alone here; there are others out there who are suffering, whose suffering is our suffering. Be kind. Give from the heart. That's all it is really about. Just be kind.

Bernie Siegel, M.D.

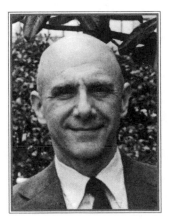

ernie Siegel, a former pediatrician and general surgeon, teaches medical professionals and patients the importance of love and positive thinking to facilitate healing. "What is lacking in the medical profession is the acceptance of people as having feelings," he says. "We need to treat the story and the life, not just the diagnosis."

The Power of Love

People are now doing research on things they used to call crazy. A study of Harvard students shows you have fewer illnesses if your parents loved you; if you are living a busy, active life, you may be exposed to more people but you have fewer colds and get sick less often; those women who have a loved one with them in the room while they are giving birth need less anesthesia and have fewer cesarean sections. We are proving that love is part of our physiology, that our feelings manifest in our body.

I was born the ugly duckling. My mother had delivery problems and I was born with great trauma to my skull and face, so I was black, blue, hemorrhaged, and distorted. It was too painful for my mother to take me out in the street because I looked like a monster. In the story, the ugly duckling's mother couldn't take it anymore, so she kicked him out and he had to discover for himself that he wasn't ugly. I had an advantage as I had a grandmother who said, "Give him to me." She took me and literally anointed my head with oil and massaged and pushed all the features back to where they belonged. All I knew was that this wonderful person picked me up three or four times a day and rubbed me. Now if you do that to kittens, they open their eyes earlier; if you do it to babies in the nursery, they gain weight faster. They just benefit from the love.

If I had one controllable public health issue, it would be to train all parents to be loving parents so that their kids could grow up and not be so destructive. Love is the most powerful weapon available to us, yet people can handle rage more easily. Identify people you've been having trouble with, call them up and give them hell, and they will scream back. But call them up and say, "I have decided to love you," and you will get silence; they won't know what to do next. You want to give it to your enemies? Love them! It doesn't mean lie down and let them walk all over you. You don't have to like them. But love them!

If I am mad at you, then you are in charge of my life. The last time this happened to me was a few years ago when somebody robbed our hotel room. I knew who it was as I had passed him in the hallway. Afterward I was waking up every day wishing I were back in that hallway, because what I would have done to him physically was not a nice thing. And that was the image I was living with until I realized he was in charge of my life: I was thinking about him every day. Then into my mind came this image of him taking all our things, pawning them, and buying presents for his children. And suddenly I had a big smile on my face. Somebody else said to me that he's probably just a drug addict and bought drugs. But every time I think of that man I just smile, and if I met him, I would say, "I've got another hundred bucks for you because I want you to be sure you get your kids some really nice things." Now I'm free of him; he doesn't bother me any more. When you feel rage, it means someone else is in charge of your life.

Love keeps me going, to be able to give it and experience it. The spiritual teachings of all the religions have told us for centuries that action, wisdom, and devotion are essential for us each to be a whole person—action, wisdom, devotion, and a fighting spirit with a willingness to change and learn. The teachings are all there in the work of the great prophets of the past. What we ought to be doing is reissuing the important books and saying to the kids, "Read this. Don't wait till you get cancer or are hit by a truck or fall out a window to discover how to survive." Whether it's an illness, a difficult relationship, a job loss, or money problems, there are ways of living, and we have already been given the instructions.

When people say, "Something has happened; I am now willing to look at my life and change," I will say, "Okay, let me be your coach. What do you want to be, what do you want to become? Who could be a role model for you? Let us work at your becoming the person you want to be." And that really sums up my therapy: find out who you want to be, then go home and practice. Practicing means it's okay to forgive yourself if you don't always get it right. I hold this role model up in front of myself and I rarely live up to it, but I forgive myself and I apologize to the people who are not receiving all the love I'd like to give them. I keep practicing and rehearsing. When you do that, then the people in your life forgive you because they know that you're trying to accomplish something and that if you fail, it just means you're human.

With every patient, there are three questions that I ask. Firstly, "What do you want for dinner?" This is to know whether they are in touch with their feelings. If they answer quickly—in five or ten seconds—they are telling me what they feel they want for dinner; they are not evaluating cost, fat content, protein, nutrition. Secondly I ask, "How would you introduce yourself to God?" When you introduce yourself to God by saying, "I don't need an introduction; I am you," then you have that worth, and that's what I'm trying to help people find. Thirdly I ask, "What do you hold up in front of the world to show everybody how beautiful and meaningful life is?" When people can say, "Hold me up, or just put a mirror in front of me," then they know they are beautiful and wonderful, and they are being guided by their feelings. We all need to realize that we have this great potential in us. It's not about failing; it's not about "Arise and walk," but it is about our sins being forgiven. Healing comes when you live a life of love and freedom from feeling like a sinner.

What people don't believe in they don't support, and so it takes time for minds to open and accept. What is lacking in the medical profession is the acceptance of people as having feelings. Most of the people who go into the medical profession have healthy reasons, but, as in many other professions, the training does not get you to look at your personality, qualities, and characteristics. Without this you can hurt the people you are caring for. They teach you about the diagnosis rather than the story, but people are living stories; they are not AIDS or cancer or multiple sclerosis. They may be in hell, burning up, or having a wake-up call. The same disease can be a gift to one person and a burden to another. We need to treat the story and the life, not just the diagnosis.

We are not taught how to deal with our feelings or the patient's feelings, so doctors suffer from post-traumatic stress disorder. If you come back from a war, you can go into therapy and deal with what you saw. But if you are working in a hospital, there are no meetings with therapists to talk about watching death and suffering and making some sense out of it all. We are not taught about our ability to heal or how attitudes affect health. It's just a mechanical training. I am not denying there are a lot of people around today who are living and loving who would not have been fifty years ago, all because of heart transplants and other technical breakthroughs, but mechanically treating people doesn't help them to heal their lives; it doesn't stop self-destructive behavior.

Everybody knows what's good for them. You could go out on the street right now and stop five people and say, "Can you answer these five questions about diet, exercise, spirituality, alcohol, and tobacco?" They'll give you the right answers, but that doesn't mean they are doing them. I know people who smoke outdoors so that their pets will not be exposed to cigarette smoke. What is that about, that they love their pets more than themselves? I go nuts seeing one commercial after another on television telling us how to avoid pain and headaches or acid problems. They don't say, "Change your life" or "Change your attitude"; they say, "Take a pill and go on doing what caused this in the first place." Nobody ever says that you might learn from your pain or that life is difficult so how can we deal with the difficulty? It's always, "Become numb or distracted, or buy this."

Twenty years ago I painted a portrait of myself in my surgical garb, and it helped me to realize how sick I was. There's a man in a cap and a gown, but you look in those eyes and you see a man who's in pain. I show it to people and say, "Do you want him to be your doctor?" And everybody laughs and says, "Are you kidding?" And I say, "That was me, and I want you to feel compassion for doctors because we're in a lot of pain, and that's why we put the wall up." Because we're hurting, we build a wall to protect ourselves. But you die behind a wall. It doesn't protect you. I was dying behind that wall. I got out of there because I knew it could kill me.

I believe that medicine will become more spiritual, as in the old days when physicians didn't have all these mechanical toys to play with, so they had to sit with people and care for them. There is the famous portrait *The Doctor,* which shows a doctor sitting in a cabin with a child who died on Christmas day, with the parents in the background. The doctor is sitting with his elbow on his knee and his chin in his hand. He's thinking next to the dying child. That's inconceivable to me. How can you do that? Why don't you hold that child? Why don't you tell the mother to come and pick him up? I hope in the future we will stop thinking so much and hold a lot more.

Statistics and thinking can help us make decisions about our treatment, but we also need to ask, "How do I feel about what my doctor has suggested to me?" If surgery is seen as a gift from God or a way of being free of a disease, you could wake up and not have any pain and leave the hospital in a few days. But if it is seen as a mutilation, then you may be there for a week or ten days in pain. If you feel, "I'm going through hell, and I don't want this, and I don't like my doctor, and I have no family caring about me," then that will affect your recovery. Doctors need to bring in the caring, the story, the personal, and that it's okay to say a prayer, to touch a patient, or to offer love and support.

There are people around us all the time, and the sad part is that we don't talk to them. If we started communicating, perhaps put an ad in the papers saying, "I'm lonely; anybody else lonely too?" it would be amazing how many people would call. If you said, "How can I love the world?" versus, "What can I get out of the world?" things would begin to happen. Try going down to the local animal shelter and asking how you can help out. Take a dog for a walk and guess how much better you'll feel. The world needs some repair work; go out and repair something and look how it helps repair you.

What I would like to hang up in every public building is a photograph of someone's internal organs. Under it would be this: "Please write down the sex, religion, and race of this person. If you are correct, you will win a million dollars." But people would say, "How can I tell? That's a picture of somebody's insides." And that's right. We're all the same color inside, so why don't we get along? God created diversity to make life interesting, but we have made the diversity something to fight about. Try choosing love, choosing compassion.

I have learned that there are four ways to solve problems: remove yourself, remove the relationship, remove the other person, or ask what love could do in this situation. And if you look at the fourth solution, which I try to do in my life, then you find healthier and more interesting solutions. It's really about finding your way of loving the world. It isn't somebody else telling you to be a plumber, doctor, mother, or violinist. You choose your way of loving the world and go do it. And since almost every occupation gets you to meet people who aren't happy, you have an opportunity to change the world and improve it. So when you meet people, bring them some joy, make fun of the craziness of life. Children with illness don't say, "I could be dead in a year." They say, "Can I have some fun today? Can I go out today?"

Life is real, and the car won't start and the roof leaks and things happen, and I always say that it is easier to be a monk in a cave and be brought two meals a day and to meditate than it is to be married and have five children, and then grandchildren. To me, that's the real test. Unless my wife came in with a gun or poisoned my supper, I would never leave her. I wrote a poem for our anniversary called "Bittersweets." No matter how much bitterness she could bring into my life, it would only teach me to be more loving. So I see life as my test on how to serve and how to be more loving, rather than how to get what I want. I don't revere anybody until they say to me, "I've been married to the same woman for forty years. We have a bunch of kids and they drive me out of my mind. I've got to pay the electric bill, my car won't start, and my roof is leaking." That's when you've made it, when you know "I am here, I am in the right place, I will experience life. If I miss the plane, I miss the plane. But who knows what will happen if I miss it. Maybe that's what our creator intended." When you've achieved that kind of letting go and freedom, that's when I would say you've made it.

What each of us needs to do is to ask ourself, "Who is my Lord? Whom do I have faith in?" Is my Lord money? Is my Lord esteem, position, what other people think? Who is the Lord over my life, who am I working for, who do I have faith in? When we have the proper Lord and work out of faith in that Lord, some wonderful things begin to happen. But each of us has to decide who we have faith in and what we are here for. Every morning I take time to be by myself and say, "What are you thinking about? What's on your mind? What's going on? What's left over? What needs to be dealt with?" In every religion they tell you to meditate, take silent time for prayer or reflection. Wherever you are, just stop and say, "Let me express my love right here and now."

Jill Purce

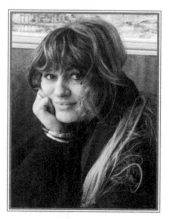

ill Purce has spent many years teaching the use of the voice through chant to heal and uplift. Here she shares how it is through resonating together that we find a deeper level of harmony and community. "To enchant means to make magical through chanting: to resonate in ourselves, to resonate ourselves with others, and to resonate with others with the Divine."

Finding Our Communal Voice

People in traditional cultures have always sung or chanted together as a part of their everyday life, whether in ceremony, at the change of the seasons, in times of celebration, or when working together. This was not something they had to be qualified for, but something they did simply to express their identity as a community, their belonging together. Traditional cultures have always understood themselves to be part of something much greater than just themselves, so singing was also a tuning together in the context of a spiritual dimension. This mutual tuning not only created a sense of community but also a sense of participating in the Divine.

In many creation stories, the voice is the vehicle for creation itself. Sound brings form into being; it transforms spirit into matter, yet at the same time it dissolves boundaries and takes matter back into spirit. We come together to chant, creating form with our presence, while the normal boundaries that separate us dissolve and we become a part of each other. This is why we have national anthems: by singing together, we become one community. Singing at football matches has the same effect; supporters unify and give energy to their team. This is a survival of the war cry, by which opposing sides created their own identity through their voices.

Chanting or singing is empowering not just spiritually and emotionally but also physically, both for individuals and for groups. Traditional chants used in this way have come to be called work songs. These were sung when people wanted to do a physical task that was greater than any one individual was able to do. When people came together to build temples or cathedrals, to bring in the crops, or to row boats from place to place, by singing together they became enormously powerful. Through the resonance of joined voices and hearts we attain an incredible ability to do things. Nowadays we have machines to do these tasks, and we no longer sing together.

With the birth of science as we know it in the seventeenth century, it began to seem more reliable to predict and control the world by measuring than by prayer and invocation. This shift in attitude from one of creating a reciprocal relationship with the Divine through chanting and praise led to our losing touch with our communal voice. More and more people now feel there is no God, and so feel no need to praise God by singing or chanting. Yet in losing our communal voice, we have lost a tremendous source of empowerment.

The chanting tradition in the church was broken in the sixteenth century; from that time Gregorian chant was lost until the nineteenth century when it was reinvented. Nobody knows whether the way it is now sung was how it used to sound, but most people think not. Yet it is a survival of what some have described as a time when we had choirs perpetually engaged in praising God. In the monasteries, the community would come together seven times a day to praise God through chanting. In between times, the members would mend the roof or work in the fields. But the aim of these communities was to perpetually praise God by chanting. Now, some of these communities have felt that instead of being invigorating, empowering, and a profound meditation, chanting is debilitating and getting in the way of more important, more pressing tasks, and so in recent years it has been gradually reduced.

Another of the contributions to our silence is a historical one and has to do with musical literacy. When we started writing music down, we were able to start creating incredibly sophisticated and complex musical pieces which became the great Western musical tradition, but in so doing, only those people who read or understood music could participate. So music became increasingly the domain of professionals, separate from that of the ordinary people who simply listened. It became less important what the effect of the sound was; it was no longer created in order to be effective, as a means to move either matter or the Spirit.

This separation from our voice is not just damaging to our spiritual health but also to our physical health, since the body itself is a resonant system. The very first thing that happens to us when fertilization occurs—when we become an individual entity—is the creation of a cell that pulsates. This pulsating cell becomes the beating heart. And so our original identity, as separate from the world, is this pulsation. As we develop, this pulsation becomes one of many, and so we have pulsations of the heart, the organs, each of the different parts of our bodies. We are full of rhythms, from the pulse of the brain to the movement of walking or dancing.

When we are ill, it is as if all these resonances have become out of tune with each other; they are no longer resonating in harmony. The first thing that chanting does is enable us to tune the different parts of ourselves together, so that we become a resonant instrument again. By tuning each of the organs, we tune our whole body; we can literally resonate the body to a state of health. As we chant, we stimulate various glands and affect our brain chemistry—stimulating endorphins and serotonin and other natural chemicals that bring about a state of calm or relaxation and a reduction of stress. This increases our overall state of well-being.

However, chant does more than heal us in a physical way. Our mental health develops in relationship to the community: when we are most healthy, we are in a resonant state with the outside world. People who commit suicide are people who are out of tune with their world. So a very important part of being healthy or healed is being in tune with our society, our community, and our family or with those with whom we are in relationship.

In addition to being healthy, we need a harmonious way of expressing our feelings; as a result of no longer chanting or singing together, we have lost a very healthy way of doing this. Unexpressed emotions can create distress, depression, or disease. When you sing, you automatically open and liberate yourself; you create flow, because there is literally a channel opening in you and you are flowing out of that channel. And if you're flowing out of that channel, something can flow into and through you. So chanting together is very important as a part of both the psychological and emotional healing processes.

One of the main causes of illness is related to how we perceive. Every time we perceive something, whether through smelling, tasting, touching, hearing, or seeing, we name it. This enables us to feel safe in the presence of something because it is known to us, it is recognized and recognizable, we have known it safely before and will know it again in the future. However, by naming it, all the associations that we have with it from before are present whenever we use the name, as are all the things we haven't done and therefore have to do in association with it. And so every perceptual act—every moment we use our senses—creates a separation between us and what we perceive and at the same time creates a regret of the past and burdens of obligation to the future. It is this cycle of anxiety that makes us so sick.

Chanting enables us to be in the present: at the same time we are chanting, we are also listening to ourselves chant, and so we cannot be thinking about what we didn't do or what we have to do; by listening to ourselves chanting while we are chanting, we become at once the chanter, the chanted, and the chant itself. Being in the present, being in the unfolding moment, is the most powerful form of healing.

Chant is a way of opening ourselves to God, of opening to other people, and also of being open to other people who are in turn being open to us. The flow of the heart can only happen between two hearts that are open. This is resonance. In particular, chanting overtones—chanting on one note in such a way that you selectively amplify the component notes or overtones of sound itself so that they become louder than the note you are singing—gives us this resonant base because we are working with the very structure of nature, its sonorous structure. We are making audible our own geometry. We resonate ourselves with the Divine structure of all things. When we chant the overtones, our internal geometries can resonate in tune with themselves. If we are constantly tuning to music that is out of tune, like the Western tempered scale, then on some level we are held in a state of distortion. When we work with the overtones, we let all the parts of our being drop into their real formations, and the body recognizes this.

We need to rediscover the traditional ways of working with the voice, not just as prayer but also as meditation. These methods are practiced in traditions with unbroken lineages, such as in the Tibetan tradition in which chant or mantra is an integral part of its meditative practice. The importance of a mantra is not that the words have a discursive meaning; on the contrary, their repetitious nature is such that the words take you beyond the discursive mind into participation with the great Mind, or the Divine. With a mantra you are also tuning into the morphic field of everyone who has ever attained enlightenment through the chanting of that mantra.

It's not surprising that we have become so disenchanted. We can only be re-enchanted if we begin chanting again, if we reconnect with our communal voice. To enchant means to make magical through chanting: to resonate in ourselves, to resonate ourselves with others, and to resonate with others with the Divine. When we open our voices, we open our hearts; the voice of the heart is the mind of compassion that is at the very center of our being.

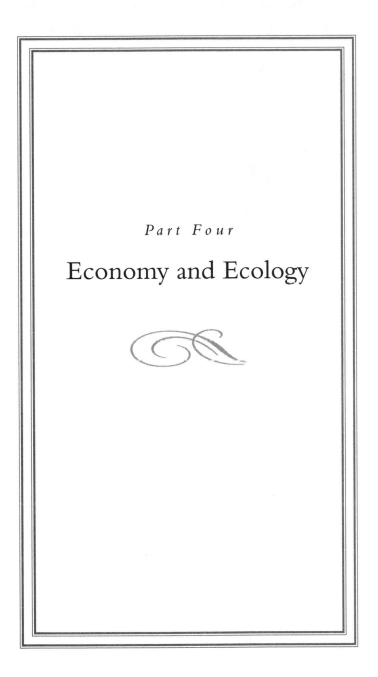

Part Four

Economy and Ecology

Muhammad Yunus

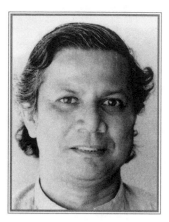

Founder of the Grameen Bank in Bangladesh, Muhammad Yunus developed the concept of microcredit and a banking system that has given millions of the most impoverished a chance to rebuild their lives and their self-esteem. "I firmly believe that all human beings have an innate survival skill," he states. "By our giving the poor people credit, they can start putting those survival skills into good use."

Microcredit

Money Does Buy Happiness

My dream is the total eradication of poverty from the world. In two to three decades from now I want my grandchildren to be able to go to museums to see what poverty was like. There is no reason why this cannot happen. There are 1.2 billion poor people in the world. Grameen Bank has so far assisted 2 million of these, while other microcredit organizations have reached a further 4 million. Given the number of dependents most of these people have, we estimate that 36 million people have so far been assisted to move above the poverty line.

If we are going to overcome poverty, then we have to rethink the whole business. We have to be revolutionary, to do things that seem impossible but actually work. Microcredit is very simple, and yet it has never been done before in a professional way. It works by helping the people individually and directly, by giving them money in the form of small personal loans, rather than the usual system of giving large sums to organizations for rural or social development. I firmly believe that all human beings have an innate survival skill. The fact that the poor are alive is the proof of this ability. We do not need to teach them how to survive; they know this well enough already. By giving them credit, we create the situation in which they can start putting those survival skills to good use.

In 1972 I was the head of the economics department at Chittagong University. Bangladesh had recently become independent and many people were desperately poor. Fifty years of international aid programs had not helped alleviate the poorest of the poor. While I was teaching the theories of economics in the privileged surroundings of an academic institution, people were dying of hunger all around us. We knew the theories of how economic development should work, but we knew nothing about real poverty or any practical way to address it. How could these people, who worked all day, still be so poor? It did not make sense. The only recourse I could find was to go to the poor people themselves to see how they lived and why it was all going wrong.

So I took my students out to the villages and for a few years we studied the lives of these people. We sponsored improved farming techniques and irrigation systems, but that did not affect the truly poor, the most destitute of all who had nothing. How could we help them? Finally, I came to understand that the problem lay in cash flow. Money that had to be borrowed to buy the materials needed for making a basket, stool, or other salable item had to be repaid at such a high rate of interest that only the most minimal profit was left— not enough to survive on. The problem was not the ineptitude of the peasants, a lack of intelligence, or laziness, but the system of agents and profit makers that dominated their lives. Some money lenders set interest rates as high as 10 percent a week. Without capital the workers had no hope; they were caught in an economic trap.

The solution lay in a credit system that the poorest of all could cope with. To try this, I lent forty-two poor people a total amount of $27. Freed from agents and merchants, the borrowers could buy their own supplies and sell their own produce, and thus double their income. Within a few days the loans were being repaid. We continued in this way, lending minimal loans to an ever-growing number of borrowers and watching them begin to make a profit for themselves.

At this point I thought how simple it would be if the major banks did this; they could open local branches and help so many people. But no such luck. The bankers thought my ideas would never work, that poor people were not trustworthy and would never repay their loans, that they were too lazy, unintelligent, and certainly not creditworthy, that they had brought on their misfortune themselves. So I continued on my own, working with ever-larger groups of borrowers, trying to prove to the banks how very trustworthy these people were. Finally, in 1979, the Central Bank agreed to fund a pilot for the Grameen Bank (which means "rural bank") with the participation of seven banks. However, in only four years the expansion rate was so fast—by then we had 59,000 borrowers—that by 1983 we decided to set up the Grameen Bank as a separate institution. Today Grameen is the biggest bank in Bangladesh with over 2 million borrowers. By 1995 it had lent more than $1.3 billion, and by 1998 it plans to lend double that amount. At the moment 92 percent of the bank's shares are owned by the borrowers themselves. By 1995, the bank made enough profit to wean itself off subsidized support from various donors.

A typical loan size is about seventy dollars. Most of the borrowers—94 percent—are women; I have found that women are far better at handling money and repaying their debts than most men are. In Bangladesh many of the women have never touched money before, are widowed or divorced or have a sick husband, and have children to feed, clothe, and educate; many have been forced into prostitution or begging in order to survive. Through the loan a woman can buy the necessary materials to make baskets or bangles, or a cow to milk and sell the produce.

Rabitan was deserted by her husband when she was six months pregnant. She had to move in with her mother who was a beggar. Rabitan had been raised by begging, and now she was being forced to beg to raise her own child. With her first Grameen Bank loan she sold bangles and earrings from door to door. Just to move away from begging was a huge achievement for her. By the end of the year she had repaid her loan, and with the second loan she expanded her business further and was able to rebuild her shack and add bamboo mat walls. With her third loan she started a stationery and grocery store in a corner of her shack. Her next goal is to get her son educated, something her mother could never have dreamed of for her daughter.

Most loans are fully repaid within a year, by which time the borrower is making a small profit and is eligible for another loan. Within a few years many are becoming independent; they are feeding their families, sending their children to school, and even buying a small piece of land to farm. They are no longer in poverty, and they have gained dignity and pride alongside financial freedom. A study by Helen Todd in 1996 showed that about 50 percent of the borrowers who have been with the Grameen Bank for more than eight years have crossed the poverty line.

When Hawa Bewa's husband died, she and her four children had to move into a rich man's house where she worked as a domestic servant. After about a year of applying for a loan, one was arranged for her. She invested the first two loans in paddy husking that generated enough savings to buy a small piece of land and to build a straw shack for her family. The third loan enabled her to lease 0.14 acre of farmland. Her eldest daughter helps her with the husking, and she hopes to soon send her two younger sons to school. Hawa now belongs to a collective of sixty people who have launched a joint enterprise of stocking paddy with a Grameen Bank loan.

In order to get a loan, the borrower has to be poor, and among the poor the very poorest get preference. We also ask any potential borrower to form a group with four other borrowers. The members of this group of five then strengthen and assist each other, giving each other discipline, mutual support, and courage. They also ensure loan repayment is in time; otherwise the entire group suffers. This has led to a 95 percent average of loan repayments, which most commercial banks would be delighted to have.

The borrowers also have to agree with the Grameen Bank basic principles, known as the "sixteen decisions," which are aimed at enabling them to improve their lives. These include:

to use discipline, unity, courage, and hard work to advance in all walks of our lives

to bring prosperity to our families

to repair our houses and work toward constructing a new home

to grow and eat more vegetables

to plant as many seedlings as possible

to keep our families small and to look after our health

to educate our children

to care for the environment

to drink clean water

not to take or give any dowry in regard to our children's marriages and not to practice child marriage

not to inflict injustice on anyone

to always be ready to help another

Obviously microloans are not an answer to all problems of poverty. Enabling an individual to become self-reliant does not deal with severe sanitation, medical, or social problems. However, helping the poorest of the poor to find their feet is an area that has long been ignored. I feel that many aid programs are only dealing with the general issues and not the individuals, making poverty bearable rather than overcoming it. Once financial support is available, and particularly in a form that stimulates the instinct to survive, then often the only major problem that impedes someone becoming financially independent is his or her state of health; through malnutrition some are just too physically infirm to help themselves.

It is encouraging to see the basic ideas of Grameen now being applied in different countries where the social and lifestyle conditions differ vastly. Microcredit banking is a means to empower people so they can create a better life for themselves and their families. In the United States there are five hundred microcredit projects in places as diverse as a ghetto in Chicago and a Native American reservation.

It has been interesting to see how in some urban communities the lack of real community—of a sense of a shared life, of care for each other, of solidarity—has hindered the process. How do we gather groups of five to work together when one will not work with even one other? This lack of community is a major impediment to overcoming poverty. However, in the shanty towns of Dhaka, 18,000 borrowers are now participating in a microcredit organization—the Shokhti Foundation; this shows that it is possible for people in urban communities to work together. The same is being seen in urban areas of India, the Philippines, and an increasing number of other countries. Overcoming poverty—raising the poor above the poverty line—can only be achieved when we work together for the benefit of all.

Anita Roddick

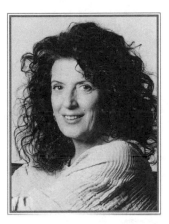

As the founder of The Body Shop, Anita Roddick has become a major voice for ethical business and environmental issues, alongside human rights and animal welfare. She states, "I see a future in which corporations empower their employees, in which the social auditing of a company is common practice. My vision for the next decade is that business is inextricably linked with the community at large."

Social Responsibility in Business

Business has as much potential to unite or destroy lives as does war. Half the world's biggest economies are corporations. Many of us in business, especially when we travel in the majority world and see the results of Western economic policies, have a rumbling disquiet about much of what our economic institutions have done. According to the free trade theory, we should be happy that the globe is becoming a playground for those who can move capital from place to place in search of the lowest wages, the most passive workers, and the loosest environmental regulations. But I have held mutilated babies, genetically handicapped by toxic wastes dumped in local streams. I have seen the damage done to communities when the big corporations suddenly move on.

However, businesses are created by humans and are therefore subject to the changes that humans impose on them. Now is the time to put some idealism back on the global agenda so that corporations become a force for positive change. A new paradigm is needed, a whole new framework for seeing and understanding this. Business must not only avoid hideous evil; it must actively do good.

This company, The Body Shop, is for profit—it is a listed company on the stock market—and yet it acts in a not-for-profit way. For instance, we have forty people working on human rights, social justice, and trading with communities in need. People can't understand our spending money like this. They do not realize that it may not have anything to do with face creams, but it has everything to do with who we are.

There are no signposts to this type of thinking, no books explaining how to run a socially responsible company, so all of what we do is experimental. To help us, we have developed two main areas of action. Firstly, we have an ethical auditing process—a systematic approach to measuring our social and environmental impact. We realized that we are not just beholden to the shareholders but we also have a whole community of people we are responsible for: we have our employees—who are our biggest responsibility—our suppliers, the communities in which we have stores, the environment that we have an impact on, the people who receive money from The Body Shop Foundation, and the people and their communities with whom we trade in the majority world. These are all stakeholders. And we ask them, "How are we meeting your needs, what are your aspirations from us, how have we screwed up, and how have we done a good job?" This is a huge, in-depth, and ongoing process. And we publish the results on this process every two years.

Secondly, we have the networking of best practices, such as exchanging ideas with Levi's on human rights issues or with Reebok on third-party manufacturing in the Far East. We talk to companies in Scandinavia as they have extraordinary good practice in business; or we look to past businesspeople such as the Quakers and see how they could run a great company while maintaining a strong relationship with the community. When you deal with subjects that are in the closet—human rights and international trade, for instance— there are no guidelines on how to use your shops to campaign or how to incorporate spirituality into the workplace. That is not in the business lexicon. Productivity is, but not productivity of the human spirit. It is uncharted territory. You tread in it, and one day it is like a landmine and another day it is like an oasis of sanity.

I know this company has got to be groundbreaking; I know it has to have a vision that we live and breathe every minute we are open for trading, every day of the year, in every country that we are in, wondering if we are being better, kinder, or more thoughtful. How are we impacting on the environment with all our manufacturing? How are we aiming toward sustainability? How are we efficient in our campaigning? How do we embrace the human spirit in a company as complex as this? I know the route to go, but the process of getting there, of making sure that it is inherent in every organizational chart and every function and assessed in every job description, is a much harder journey. This is especially true when we have the traditional disciplines of manufacturing, quality control, distribution, and marketing to maintain.

There is a lot of reflection in the self-realization movement, but unless it is translated into social justice, it is wasted. So how do we translate it? I have always believed that the personal becomes the political and the political becomes the global; it is not possible to run a business without involving the politics of consciousness in some way. One of the hardest things that we need to achieve is a global perspective that embraces a sense of responsibility. Obviously we cannot stop business from going global, but we can make it listen to the responsibilities that go with the territory. We must know the results of the decisions we make on the environment and the community. Business should not be using the planet as a pit-stop race to the bottom, in which it just looks for the most docile workers and the cheapest labor conditions, in countries where human rights abuse runs rampant and where toxic wastes and bitter communities are left behind when the business moves on and everything is closed down.

I do not think this can come from government regulations. It has to come from businesses' realizing that acting responsibly and responsively is good for them. I see a future in which corporations empower their employees, in which the social auditing of a company is common practice. My vision for the next decade is that business is inextricably linked with the community at large. Business cannot avoid moral choices; its future depends on them.

There are a growing number of companies that think like us. We belong to informal associations like Business for Social Responsibility and Social Venture Network in which we share ideas. We have "circles of innovation" in which ten to fifteen companies come together to discuss ideas and to see how each other works. We encourage each other to implement a growth in social responsibility. This is about how we manage our waste, how we clean up our mess, how we minimize energy use. Often, with thinking like this, we have got to be the first ones with a toe in the water. And then others say, "Oh, that's not too bad. You are still profitable. We can play along with that."

But what we need more than anything is emotional support because the media often have a go at us, especially the financial journalists. It would be so much easier to run a skin- and hair-care company in which we put millions of pounds into an ad campaign that says, "You really need this to make yourself sexier." Doing that is a no-brainer. Being socially responsible is not easy. Whenever the financial press measures a company by its share price or profits, I ask, "Profit for whom? What about how a company profits emotionally?"

In the same way that we deny the spirit in business, so the cosmetics and media industries have turned aging into a disease. It's very, very clever. If you are in constant need of repair, then there has to be something to repair it; and the way to repair it is by looking at an image that tells you what you should be like, alongside the products that will do this. Aging is a billion-dollar industry. Part of the mythology of the cosmetics industry is that every moisture cream works. The huge success of antiaging creams baffles me because it doesn't take a rocket scientist to realize there is no way you can put a mixture of water and oil (which is all creams are) on your body and—whoosh!—your breasts are augmented or your thighs get thinner or you take away twenty years of environmental degradation. It can't be done. In the windows of our shops we had a poster that said, "The only way to avoid wrinkles is to never smile again," either that or you must live in space.

The aging process has become one of diminishment in beauty rather than one of growing in wisdom. In the Gabra tribe in East Africa, older women are considered more sensual because they carry greater wisdom. Young men learn wisdom from older women, while older men aspire to be as a woman: men in their sixties and seventies spend time with women, dress as women, weave and tell stories with women. They don't need antiaging creams to make them more beautiful.

The energy of activism is my spirit and soul. I think immigrants are always marginalized, and we were the only Italian family living in a small town. We also had a very outraged mother who hated the Catholic Church and yet sent us dutifully to convent school. She squashed garlic on our fingers every Sunday and sent us to church to "pollute" it with the smell; or she sent us to school in trousers and the nuns sent us back to put on skirts, so we were like yo-yos. She challenged everything. Without her knowing it, she put us on the edge of bravery all the time. I stood on street corners collecting money for Freedom from Hunger or marched for the Campaign for Nuclear Disarmament. I hadn't a clue what any of these things were about; I just knew I had to be brave and challenge the system.

For five months of the year I get out of the office, out of the chair, and I usually travel toward people who have a stronger vision than I have. Traveling has grounded me in the most fundamental of insights: that all life is an expression of a single spiritual unity; that we are not, as humans, on top of anything but we are instead a part of everything. This interconnection has to be sacred, reverent, and respectful of all ways of knowing and being. I traveled in the rural Black Belt of the United States with a vagabond, through Mississippi and Alabama and Georgia. I lived in the communities in shacks, and I looked at the role of crack and the entrepreneurship of drug dealing. I saw the role of the mother diminishing as she is now making and selling the stuff, and the role of the grandmother growing because she is pivotal in trying to maintain values and care, and I saw that there is structured racism holding that society in place.

Such experiences shape my values as a business leader. I go mostly to see if there is a way, perhaps through a small-scale economic initiative, that can keep a community together. But I also go for fear of losing a sense of empathy with the human condition. When your values are embedded in a very working-class Italian family and then you receive wealth through your work, it can corrode you. Wealth can separate you from the human condition. That fear of separation makes me maintain these hugely important reality checks. The only skill that I have to share is trading, and it comes through projects that we fund. These projects do not focus on the financial reports, but a company like ours should be measured by how it treats the weak and the frail, rather than how profitable we are or how large our market share is.

So, for example, in Australia we helped set up a playground dedicated to visually and mentally handicapped kids, which was a young staff member's vision. The Body Shop donated seed money, Perth 200 donated the land, and then we managed to knock on doors and get the Variety Club of Western Australia to donate the remaining funds required; and this extraordinary playground is in place. I work with community projects, like Childhope in the Philippines, and we go into the communities of street children. Childhope uses little pedicabs that have visual aid material inside, and it gives the kids information, education, and help. In Glasgow, in probably the worst housing area in Western Europe, we set up a factory which employs about 120 people making soap and which puts back into the community a certain percentage of the money generated. It has funded a children's adventure playground, a place for handicapped people, a home for women who have suffered domestic violence, and so on.

We work with Human Rights Watch around the world and fund their offices in Brussels and in Bosnia. We have given around a million dollars' worth of funding to date. Also everyone who works for us has the opportunity to do half a day a month in local community service. In both Brixton and Harlem we operate community shops in which a percentage of the stores' profits goes back to the local community. The stores do some fabulous projects, ranging from working with people with AIDS to maintaining homes for those who have suffered domestic violence to running literacy programs. Each shop chooses what it wants to do.

The knowledge that I have gained as an entrepreneur is that we have to have a vision of something new; we have to believe in something so strongly that it becomes a reality. One of the campaigns we did was with Amnesty International to help release prisoners of conscience. We had posters in shops and we got signatures and wrote letters, and then we heard that some prisoners had been released. When a member of your staff looks you straight in the eye and puts her hands on your shoulders and says, "This is the real me," you know she's not going home and dreaming of moisture creams. She's going home and dreaming of how she is able to help, how she can challenge the system and change the status quo. Enthusiasm, when it comes straight from the heart, is unbelievable in terms of its energy. It is unstoppable.

I think we'll look back in a couple of decades and wonder what the nineties did. Maybe the nineties was about transformation. You know, that time when the chrysalis gets very messy and then it changes into a butterfly? It's messy, it's putrid, it's yeuch! And yet that process is so creative. The end of every millennium has always been more reflective, more responsible and creative; revolutions always come at the beginning or end of something. I hope this decade is about rethinking, in which we challenge the status quo, challenge the mechanistic way of doing things, challenge science and technology, and start talking about wisdom, magic, and spirituality, about the deeper meanings of things.

I saw a quote by Mahatma Gandhi in a really old community bank in India, addressed to people starting a new business. It said: "Look into the eyes of the poorest man or woman and ask, 'Is your work going to make his or her life any better?'" We've got to have an education that measures the morality of our behavior. We've got to have politicians who ask, "Is this the right thing to do?" We've got to have media that have a sense of social responsibility and are not all sex and violence but thoughtful, dissenting, and educating with information. I believe we should be setting up experiential and educational projects in which we talk about the production and shaping of the human spirit, rather than polishing people for a job.

We have to rethink our approach to business. And then we have to act to bring sustainable and healthy growth across the globe. We need trade which respects and supports communities and families, which encourages the education of children and the healing of the sick, which values the work of both men and women and respects human rights, which builds local economic capacities and independence, and which safeguards the environment. The underlying catastrophe is poverty—economic poverty, spiritual poverty, and poverty of the imagination.

We should challenge everything. Everything you have been taught at school, challenge it; everything you have been taught at home, challenge it. I have always lived by being courageous; it is the only place left uncrowded. There's something so vibrant and gutsy about courage; just do it.

George Bernard Shaw said, "I want to be used up when I die, for the harder I work the more I live. Life is no brief candle. To me it is a sort of splendid torch which I've got to hold up for the moment, and I want to make it burn as brightly as possible before handing it on to future generations."

Paul Hawken

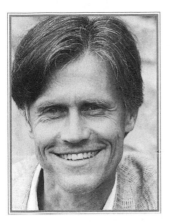

The founder of Smith & Hawken, Paul Hawken shows how sustainability is not only essential for our future but can be directly profit making. As chairman of The Natural Step, he advises businesses and governments on achieving a sustainable future. In this piece he explores the inevitability of change. "A large-scale change in society with respect to the relationships among living systems is inevitable," he states. "The challenge is, will it occur by default or by design?"

Redesigning the World

All living systems on Earth are in decline, and the rate at which they are declining is speeding up. But we cannot solve the problem within the framework that created it. It's very easy to make others wrong, and it's particularly easy to make corporations wrong because they do so much, so badly, so often. It's almost like shooting sitting ducks. What is difficult is to imagine how to get out of the situation we're in right now in a time frame that is in line with the rate of deterioration that we're seeing. A large-scale change in society with respect to living systems and the relationships among living systems is inevitable. The challenge is, how will it occur and in what manner? Will it occur by default or by design?

The mind that looks at the world in terms of design is the mind of intention. In the case of business, it is intention by default. Nobody takes credit for the industrial system that exists in the world today; nobody raises her or his hand and says, "I designed this." Suppose you said to a group of brilliant designers, "I would like you to design a system in which you have prosperity but people can't work, a system in which you emit billions of tons of pollutants into the air, which has one billion people unemployed who want to work, and which puts into living systems 70,000 chemicals invented since World War II, the effects of which we do not understand and never will understand; and I want you to do this in a way that polarizes the rich and the poor and causes increasing disparities in terms of income distribution in the world and which wastes most of the resources it uses and is only about 1 or 2 percent efficient while the other 99 percent of the resources ends up as molecular and solid waste in landfills, in the air, in the water, in bones, in mothers' milk, and in human beings. Could you do that?" Nobody could design such a system, and yet that is what we have done.

The question then arises, what if we think about this as a design problem, in other words as an artist would look at it, as opposed to an industrial problem or an environmental, social, or economic problem—all of which it is? What if we look at it artistically?

As artists and designers, we would want to meet the needs of the people in the world whose needs are not being met and the needs of the people yet to come. We would want to radically reduce the amount of energy materials we use in the next forty or fifty years, and we would have to do all this in such a way that people would see the outcome as being better than what we have today; otherwise they wouldn't do it. Not only would we have to reduce the throughput dramatically, we would also have to do it in such a way that we would offer meaningful and dignified work, not only to the one billion people in the world who cannot work but to the many people who have work which is undignified or lacks meaning and which does not pay family wages.

So that is the design opportunity that has been given to this generation. And I would like to suggest not only that it is possible but that the rudiments of that transition are already in place and can be discerned and seen. This is a transition away from the obsessive and maniacal, although understandable, pursuit of industrialism, which is a movement designed to increase human productivity. That is what the industrial age did so magnificently. It was a huge success on that level; we should applaud it, have speeches and give it gold watches, and then retire it and send it home, because it's over.

What we have today is an abundance of human beings, but we are losing the services of our natural capital, our natural resource systems, and our ecosystems. They are declining. So we have an economy that is completely upside down and backward, because as we make people more productive, we need fewer of them. What we need to do is make our resources more productive so we need less of them. And we want to do that in such a way that we need more people. The only way that we can create a transition that moves toward radical resource productivity is to create a system that requires more human beings, not fewer. Whether it's farming or timber or a complex, closed-loop industrial system with technical nutrient cycles, we want a system that needs more people and less stuff, not more stuff and fewer people.

This transition is one in which we are moving from an economy that emphasizes human productivity to one that emphasizes resource productivity. In order to do this, we have to change our mental maps. We are trying to use old mental maps to solve new problems. Changing them is difficult, because most people's mental maps are established by education, by their peers, and by corporations.

Shared mental models are extremely important for any society. Without them we cannot drive on our roads; we have a shared mental model of what traffic is. We can't have a football match unless both teams and, for that matter, all spectators have a shared mental model of how many people play, what the goals are, what the rules are, and how long it lasts. When we, as a people, have a shared mental model, we can do magnificent things, like put an electric car on the moon. But we cannot put an electric car in Los Angeles as we do not have a shared mental model of Los Angeles.

So, for a society to move in a way that takes advantage of the differences and the diversity of expertise, knowledge, and experience that we, its members, share, we need a shared mental model that makes sense. Right now, essentially we have a system in which there is no shared framework of understanding. It is emblematic that we have mental models for football and golf but we have no mental model, no shared framework or user's manual, for the most important system of all, Earth.

There are several mental models that are now emerging. One is Factor 10, which says we can and must over the next forty to fifty years reduce the throughput of materials in the North by 90 percent. It looks at the existing system and says we can reduce the throughput right now by 70 to 80 percent with no new technologies, and we can go ahead toward 90 percent in the next forty to fifty years. We have to do this if we have a shred of compassion for ourselves or for others. Much of the resources we are using are desperately needed by other people, who do not have the privilege of buying the environment, wasting it, and then sending it back to the land as garbage. Most people in the world need to be better taken care of, and we cannot offer any means to do that unless we understand better how to take care of ourselves. What we are talking about is becoming 10 to 15 percent more resource efficient in the next forty to fifty years. I think we can do that.

Another shared framework that is emerging, that has deep intellectual roots in Germany, is what's called extended product responsibility or a take-back system. This says that we have to make our processing and manufacturing techniques mimic natural systems, because in nature there is no such thing as waste in a dynamic sense: all waste equals food for living systems. A product typology is being started. It is now being legislated step by step in Sweden, Holland, Germany, Austria, and Japan, and is beginning a little bit on a voluntary basis in the United States. It means that if someone makes something, such as a TV, a refrigerator, a VCR, or a car, then that thing belongs to the manufacturer forever. The customer only buys the use of it, and when he or she is done with it, he or she takes it to a deshopping center. It goes back to the manufacturer, and there are no more landfills. In other words, the manufacturer has to design it so that waste equals nutrients for a future production cycle.

What "take-back" legislation is saying is that there are three types of products you can make in the world: consumables, service products, and unsalables. These terms were first coined by Michael Braungart and Justus Englefried. Consumables are things that, literally, if you place them on the land, they will decompose into food for organisms with no deleterious effects. You may say, "That's easy. Wool, cotton, and silk all come from nature; we can place them on the compost pile." But when you start to analyze what we do to our natural products, you find that in fact they are not so natural at all. For instance, some black clothing is fixed with mordants containing heavy metals, so when you see those advertisements that say "Nothing comes between me and my Calvins," be aware that there are actually about 7,000 chemicals that come between you and your Calvins.

We are making things, but where are we going to put them when we are done? A landfill? Lined with plastic that is guaranteed not to leak for twenty years? Molecules will always go back into living systems, so this typology is saying that if it's not consumable, then it's a service product. What the manufacturer is selling is the service of that product, and when the buyer is done with it, is the manufacturer's again. The manufacturer has to take it back; it cannot, in the night, ship the used product out across the border to a landfill in another country. This is creating not only a design revolution but a revolution in molecular chemistry. Companies are literally discovering what it is that they make now that they are looking at the prospect of its coming back in through the door, and they are realizing that it is hazardous or toxic and may kill their workers. The point of all this is to try to get designers and industry to realize that in order to move toward sustainability, they have to design products that are not just to be recycled in a downcycling mode but to be remanufactured into useful products so that we close the material loop altogether.

The third category is unsalables, which means products that should never be sold at all, like radioactivity and persistent bioaccumulative compounds. If companies sell these things, they have to tag them molecularly. That is, they have to put their name on them. So if I find DCBP in my well—a very volatile but very persistent soil fumigant that was once used—I can take it to my county agent who will be able to tell me that it has Hooker Chemical written on it. I can telephone Hooker Chemical and say, "Funny thing, I was testing my water and there is something in here that belongs to you. Would you come and get it?" We know this is true with our dogs, yet somehow we have allowed our companies to make and disperse compounds that will last literally 10,000 years in marine environments. What we are talking about is product responsibility.

Another mental model is The Natural Step, which originated in Sweden and is now in nine countries. It was started by a doctor, Karl-Henrik Robèrt, who despaired, as I think we all have at one time or another, at the constant adversarial nature of the debate within society about the environment. As a pediatric oncologist, he had children with, in many cases, incurable cancers. The children often handled it better than the parents, who could not, understandably, cope with the loss of their child. Almost to a person they would say that they would give up their life or a part of their life, organs, or anything to save the life of their child. And yet he would see those same people go out and vote for new freeways or act in a way that was destroying the world for their children's children. The question is, why is there this difference between how the group thinks and what we do as individuals?

Dr. Robèrt went to his fellow scientists and colleagues and asked them a very simple question: "What is it that we agree on? We can see what we disagree on, which is practically everything, but is there anything which we, as geologists, chemists, economists, biologists, toxicologists, epidemiologists, medical doctors, and physicists, agree on?" He wrote a paper and sent it to fifty scientists, and they sent it back. He did this twenty-one times until they had come down to a very basic description of this nonlinear, self-organizing system called Earth. Out of that emerged The Natural Step, which is a nonprofit organization that teaches corporations, municipalities, and schools the basic system conditions for sustainability. It creates a very simple shared mental model arrived at by consensus-based science. It is used as a way of discerning how they should move their professions, companies, and institutions step by step toward sustainability. You cannot collaborate as a group unless you have a shared mental model. Three-quarters of the population of Sweden lives in cities that use The Natural Step as a way to organize their ecomunicipalities.

All around the world new mental models are emerging of how we should relate to living systems. The relationship is changing. We know that the more human-made capital we make, the more cars, roads, buildings, high-rises, and TVs that we produce, the less natural capital we have. It's very simple; the richer we get, the poorer we get. We can deal with this now and do something pro-actively, as designers, or we can just wait and do it by default. Throughout the world, people are addressing this issue of industrial metabolism: how can we redesign industrial systems so that they start to conduct themselves in a way that has a dynamic relationship with the capacity of living systems to support life on Earth?

There are some who think that this is fools' work and that we should just get rid of all corporations. But corporations are here. The most disturbing thing about large, destructive multinational corporations is that they are us. It's not them; it's us. We're in this together. It's very different from the simplistic view of the world in which there are the good guys who have to convince the bad guys that they are wrong. It doesn't work that way. If you go into any room or to any group of people, anywhere in the world, and you ask the people there the one question, "How many of you woke up this morning with the intention of destroying the world?" nobody will raise his or her hand. That's how you know it's a design problem.

Most of the corporations of the world feel the pressure to change. But the chief executive officers will tell you, "I will do as much as I can to move toward change, but if I falter in my corporation's growth, I'm out of here, and the person who replaces me may not be receptive to your ideas." So one of the things you have to provide for them is a picture of growth that does the opposite in terms of impact, that is, a picture of something that can only grow if it dramatically reduces the throughput of material. They think this is unimaginable. They think, "Don't we need more stuff if business is going to grow? We sell stuff, and if we're going to grow, we need more stuff. So how can you help me?"

But it is possible. There is a large trucking company in Sweden. As you can imagine, it would normally grow by shipping more things farther distances; it has a vested interest in highways and carbon and in inefficiency. What it has done, after it was trained in The Natural Step, is create a parallel business to help companies and governments not ship at all. It sees a company shipping tomatoes one way, and another shipping them the other way. It has seen this for years, but it was never able to benefit from its knowledge. Now it sells its expertise and helps companies ship less, so it is reversing the process.

Another company in the United States, Interface, the largest commercial manufacturer of carpet tiles, is going to completely closed loop systems. It is redesigning its carpeting. The problem with reusing carpeting is that it has a backing that is polyvinyl chloride (PVC) and a facing that is nylon. Put them together and it's garbage. You can only recycle it into a bumper strip or a park bench. That's called downcycling because you can't make it into carpeting again.

What Interface is trying to do is design carpeting that is in two pieces. They fit together, but they are separate. The nylon can be depolymerized and repolymerized, and the backing can be remelted and reused.

Essentially what Interface is saying is that within this next decade it will be buying no more raw materials whatsoever. Its future raw materials will be in the landfills and on floors. Not only is it committed to doing this and moving toward it, it is being increasingly patronized by architects and others because they're doing this. Its competitors are looking at it and saying, "This company is growing and using less material." In 1996 Interface grew 20 percent and used the same amount of material it used the year before. It has said publicly that it will use less material every year, per unit of production. It has committed to that as a corporate goal.

A story was told to me about a schoolteacher who teaches art. She asked her students to draw something they love. The third-graders thought about it for a while, and then she asked them one by one what they were going to draw. She asked the first student what he was going to draw, and he said, "A picture of my home." Then she asked the next student, and he said, "I'm going to draw a picture of my mother." Then she asked Mary what she was going to draw, and Mary piped up very cheerily, "I'm going to draw a picture of God." And the teacher got very uncomfortable and her face sort of got scrunched up, and she said, "But Mary, we don't know what God looks like." And Mary said, "No, but you will when I've finished my drawing."

I would suggest that we are all Mary, that we all design this world that we live in, that it is in need of radical redesign, and that what we are on the threshold of is completely reimagining and redesigning every single thing which we do, which we make, which we create, which we offer, which we serve to each other. Nothing will remain the same as we understand it today. We, like Mary, do not know what we are drawing, but we had better be like Mary, in the sense that we go ahead. We don't have antecedents, we don't have mentors, we only have each other. And we have an embodied, deep-seated faith that we have the design templates around us everywhere, every day, and they are nature and natural living systems.

Helena Norberg-Hodge

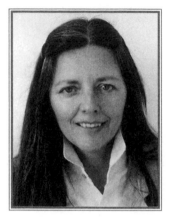

For more than twenty years Helena Norberg-Hodge has been involved with the people of Ladakh, where she has witnessed the effect of Westernization and globalization on a small, remote tribal land. A strong and powerful voice in favor of localization, she argues that "the global economy is so destructive precisely because it is attempting to hold still an evolutionary process: the dialogue between living human beings and a living biosphere."

Gaia Versus the Global Village

Why is it that everything we hold dear seems threatened? Why do we feel insecure in our working lives, in our neighborhoods and streets, even within our own homes? Why, in spite of massive public awareness campaigns and educational efforts, does the environment continue to deteriorate from year to year? Why are communities and families fragmenting, while ethnic conflict, poverty, violence, and crime are continuing to grow? Why is democracy slipping away?

If each of these problems is viewed as separate and unconnected, solving all of them can easily appear impossible; being faced with a never-ending litany of seemingly unrelated problems can be overwhelming. Finding the points at which they converge can, however, make our strategy to tackle them more effective since the potential for real and lasting solutions expands enormously. A more holistic or systematic analysis reveals that the great majority of today's social and environmental crises are but symptoms of the same underlying cause: a highly centralized, global system of production and distribution—one that transforms unique and intelligent individuals into ignorant mass consumers, homogenizes diverse cultural traditions, and destroys wilderness and biodiversity, all in the name of a "global village."

The coming of this "global village" has been hailed as the dawning of a new utopia, where all peoples will live in harmony, united with one another in a borderless world of free trade. However, we must not mistake the "one world" rhetoric of globalization for the one world of Gaia, the living Earth. The "global village" connotes a supermodern world in which interdependence means being tightly linked by transport and communications infrastructure; this "village" is part of an emerging global monoculture that pays no heed to the diversity and richness of living ecosystems. Gaia's interdependence, on the other hand, refers to the unity of all life, the inextricable web in which nothing can claim completely separate or static existence.

Today, global economic development is fragmenting us and our communities, furthering our dependence on large-scale economic structures and technologies. These economic policies have led to the growth of huge multinational corporations which now dominate world trade. Many of these corporations have grown so large they outstrip governments in size and power: fifty of the one hundred largest economies in the world are not countries but corporations. Accountable to no electorate, these bodies wield enormous economic power. Five hundred corporations now control 70 percent of total world trade; just six of them control 100 percent of world trade in the staples of rice, wheat, and maize. Due to "free trade" treaties like the General Agreement on Tariffs and Trade (GATT) and the North American Free Trade Agreement (NAFTA), such corporations can easily move their operations to countries where taxes and labor costs are low and environmental regulations weak. Corporations are often lured with free land, tax breaks, and government assistance; their sheer size and financial power allow them to extract price breaks from suppliers. On such an uneven playing field, how can a local grocer possibly hope to compete against a large supermarket chain? Is it any surprise that with each year the number of small businesses, shopkeepers, and independent farmers continues to plummet?

One result of these subsidies, for example, is that the prices of mass-produced goods transported halfway round the world are artificially cheap compared with local goods. This has been particularly true in food production. It explains why apples shipped from New Zealand can displace French apples in the markets of Paris and why the shops in Mongolia, a country with twenty-five million milk-producing animals, carry more European than local dairy products on their shelves. In Spain, for instance, in small villages in Andalucia, until a few years ago you could buy a whole range of products that were from the region: all types of fruits, grapes, figs, olives, olive oil, goat cheese, and meat from local animals: a particular type of black pig thrived on these hills, so a local delicacy was dried ham from pigs fed on the acorns from the cork oak forests. The diet was diverse, but it was limited to the products that could be produced in that environment. Now, as Andalucia has become more developed, the local products in village shops are becoming very expensive and are usually sold only to the tourists. Instead one finds the packaged, standard food of the global monoculture: Nestlé's milk, instant coffee, Kellogg's Corn Flakes, Coca-Cola products, and Spam instead of the local dried ham. The food is becoming ever more processed, and it is transported from farther and farther away.

Economic globalization is affecting us all, as individuals, families, and communities, and it is putting the biosphere itself under increasing strain, leading to:

- Erosion of democracy: Even in normally democratic countries the influence of the individual is shrinking as decision making becomes centralized in supranational bodies like the European Commission, the World Bank, and the World Trade Organization.

- Global dependence: Tied to a complex system of imports and exports, countries are becoming ever more tightly linked to a volatile global economy over which they possess little or no control.

- Loss of social support: Governments are encouraged to cut back on social spending while increasing funds for the expansion of trade and industry; this enhances international competitiveness.

- Urbanization: The globalization of the economy is leading to a massive population shift from rural areas to cities. It is estimated that by 2025 over 60 percent of the world's population will live in urban centers. This is synonymous with a host of problems, such as overcrowding, unemployment, poverty, poor sanitation, and pollution.

- Undermining food security: Global commodity market structures and subsidies minimize returns to small farmers while maximizing returns to corporate intermediaries.

- Growing gap between rich and poor: Economic globalization is leading to a widening gap between haves and have-nots, both between the countries of the North and South and within the individual countries. Already the wealth of just 350 billionaires equals the annual income of the poorest 45 percent of the world's population.

- Environmental breakdown: Globalization intensifies the already serious ecological consequences of industrialization. In addition to polluted air and water and growing piles of toxic waste and nuclear debris, we face the danger of climate change from deforestation, ozone depletion, and global warming.

- Loss of cultural diversity: The earth's cultural diversity is being replaced with a uniform Western monoculture. People around the world are bombarded by media and advertising images that present the Western consumer lifestyle as the ideal, while implicitly denigrating indigenous traditions.

The Death of Diversity: The End of Evolution

People often talk about globalization as if it were the next step in evolution and the natural result of economic efficiency. It is vital to be aware that, on the contrary, globalization is a consciously planned process—a process in which treaties such as the Uruguay round of GATT, NAFTA, and currently the Multilateral Agreement on Investment (MAI) are steadily eroding our elected governments' power in favor of transnational corporations. Globalization is far from a natural process; it is occurring because governments and industries are actively promoting and subsidizing it.

We now have a perverse situation in which human beings try to clone sheep or reverse aging through modern technology, but the same people think it is not possible to stop an economic treaty because it is inevitable and "evolutionary." It is a complete reversal of reality to think that we can manipulate and control the natural world but be incapable of changing the human-made, policy-made culture of globalization. I would argue that the global economy is so destructive precisely because it is attempting to hold still an evolutionary process: the dialogue between living human beings and a living biosphere. Instead of being evolutionary, globalization is antievolution.

The most profound impact of globalization and its attendant monoculture is on the third world, where much of the world's remaining cultural diversity is to be found. In the South the majority still live rurally, partly connected through a local economy unique to their environments and available resources. Because of pressures from globalization, locally adapted forms of production are being replaced by systems of industrial production that are ever more divorced from natural cycles. In agriculture—the mainstay for rural populations throughout the South—this means a centrally managed, chemical-dependent system designed to deliver a narrow range of transportable foods for the world market.

In the process, farmers are replaced by energy- and capital-intensive machinery. As the vitality of rural life declines, villagers are rapidly being pulled into squalor in shanty towns. The Chinese government, for example, is planning for the urban population to increase by 440 million people in the next twenty years—an explosion that is several times the rate of overall population growth. Development not only pushes farmers off the land; it also centralizes job opportunities and political power in cities, and so intensifies the economic pull of urban centers.

The inner, psychological effects of development for the South are no less profound and destructive. Advertising and media images exert powerful psychological pressure to seek a better, "more-civilized" life, one based on increased consumption. But since jobs are scarce, only a fraction succeeds. The majority end up dispossessed and angry, living in slums in the shadow of advertisements for the American Dream. In this situation those on the bottom rungs of the economic ladder are at a great disadvantage. The gap between rich and poor widens, and anger, resentment, and conflict increase. This is particularly true when people from many differing ethnic backgrounds are being pulled into cities where they are cut off from their communities and cultural moorings and where they face ruthless competition for jobs and the basic necessities of life.

Individual and cultural self-esteem are eroded by the pressure to live up to the media stereotypes of blonde, blue-eyed, and clean. As a consequence, women around the world use dangerous chemicals to lighten their skin and hair, and the demand for blue contact lenses is growing in markets from Bangkok to Nairobi to Mexico City. Many Asian women even undergo surgery to make their eyes look more Western.

Contrary to the claims of its promoters, a centrally planned global economy does not bring harmony and understanding to the world by erasing the differences between us. Uprooting people from rural communities by selling them an unattainable urban white dream is instead responsible for a dramatic increase in anger and hostility, particularly among young men. In the intensely demoralizing and competitive situation they face, differences of any kind become increasingly significant, and ethnic and racial violence are the inevitable results.

My twenty-three years of experiences in Ladakh and in the kingdom of Bhutan have made me painfully aware of this connection between the global economy and ethnic conflict. In Ladakh, a Buddhist majority and a Muslim minority had lived together for six hundred years without a single recorded instance of group conflict. In Bhutan, a Hindu minority had coexisted peacefully with a slightly larger number of Buddhists for an equally long period. In both cultures, just fifteen years' exposure to outside economic pressures resulted in ethnic violence that left many people dead. In these cases it was clearly not the differences between people that led to conflict but the erosion of their economic power and identity. If globalization continues, the escalation of conflict and violence will be unimaginable; globalization means the undermining of the livelihoods and cultural identities of the majority of the world's people.

Engaged Responses to Globalization

The challenge for us, then, is to apply our principles and spiritual teachings, often developed many centuries ago in an age of localized social and economic interactions, to the highly complex and increasingly globalized world in which we now live. This means fully understanding the subtleties of both the teachings and our current situation. Spiritual teachings can sometimes be misinterpreted: the law of karma can be used to rationalize the gap between rich and poor, or even the destruction of the environment, and Christian love can lead to tolerance toward exploitative systems or institutions. Individuals are often well intentioned and should always be shown tolerance and compassion. However, it is vital that we do not confuse human beings with systems.

The global reach of the industrial culture means that it is possible to follow all the precepts of one's spiritual belief—be a good Christian or a good Buddhist or follow one's own moral promptings—while supporting exploitation and violence on the other side of the world. The centralized global economy which we are all increasingly dependent on prevents us from being intelligent, moral beings. For instance, every time we shop in the supermarket, we may be unwittingly contributing to a whole range of problems from cruelty to animals and pesticide poisoning to the pollution of drinking water and exploitation of workers. By remaining ignorant of the larger economic systems of which we are a part, we are preventing ourselves from fulfilling our potential to live humane, compassionate lives.

Changing the direction of the global economy will not be as difficult or expensive as allowing it to continue. It is heartening to realize that even the tiniest change in policy toward diversifying economic activity at the local and national levels reaps enormous systemic rewards. For instance, a more localized transport system gives tremendous benefits from the creation of jobs to a healthier environment and a more equitable distribution of resources. Similarly, support for small-town or farmers markets helps to revitalize both the cities and the agricultural economy of the surrounding regions, while reducing the money spent to process, package, transport, and advertise food.

Already, without help from government or industry, people are starting to change the economy from the bottom up. This process of localization has begun spontaneously, in countless communities all around the world. In many towns, for example, community banks and loan funds have been set up, thereby increasing the capital available to residents and businesses and allowing people to invest in their local community. In other communities, "buy-local" campaigns are helping locally owned businesses to survive even when pitted against heavily subsidized corporate competitors. These campaigns not only help to keep money from leaking out of the local economy but also help educate people about the hidden costs to jobs, to the community, and to the environment in purchasing cheaper but distantly produced products.

In some communities, Local Exchange and Trading Systems (LETS) have been established as organized, large-scale bartering systems. People list the services or goods they have to offer and the amount they expect in return. Their account is credited for goods or services they provide to other LETS members, and they can use those credits to purchase goods or services from anyone else in the system. Thus, even people with little or no money can participate in and benefit from the local economy. LETS schemes have sprung up in the United Kingdom (where there are over 250 in operation), Ireland, Canada, France, Argentina, the United States, Australia, and New Zealand.

The systems allow for the exchange of a wide range of services— carpentry, car repair, baby-sitting, sewing, school tuition, house-painting, accounting, health care, legal assistance—as well as locally produced goods and farm products. LETS systems have been particularly beneficial in areas with high unemployment. In Birmingham, England, where unemployment hovers at 20 percent, the city government has been a cosponsor of a highly successful LETS scheme. These initiatives have psychological benefits that are just as important as the economic benefits: a large number of people who were once unemployed, and therefore felt useless, are becoming valued for their skills and knowledge.

One of the most exciting and important grassroots efforts is the worldwide movements that links urban consumers directly with farmers. In some cases, consumers purchase an entire season's produce in advance, sharing the risk with the farmer. In others, shares of the harvest are purchased in monthly or quarterly installments. Consumers usually have a chance to visit the farm where their food is grown, and in some cases their help on the farm is welcomed. While small farmers linked to the industrial system continue to fail every year at an alarming rate, this movement is allowing small-scale diversified farms to thrive in growing numbers. Such initiatives have spread rapidly throughout Europe, North America, Australia, and Japan. In the United States, the number has climbed from only 2 in 1986 to 200 in 1992 and is closer to 1,000 today.

These and countless other initiatives around the world are a reflection of a growing awareness, a realization that it is far more sensible to depend on our neighbors and the living world around us than to depend on a global economic system built of technology and corporate institutions. Faced with this reality, we have little choice but to become engaged, to challenge the economic structures that are creating and perpetuating suffering the world over. We cannot claim to be spiritual beings and simultaneously support structures that are so antithetical to life itself. Uniting the personal and the political strengthens and empowers us each step of the way and takes us on a journey of interdependent self-discovery as we start experiencing the joy of being both embedded in community and connected to the natural world.

Mikhail Gorbachev

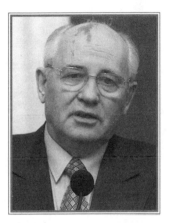

As president of the Soviet Union, Mikhail Gorbachev brought enormous social transformation through peristroika and glasnost—an openness to political affairs not seen before in Russia. In this personal account he talks about his own journey and beliefs. "Life has value in itself," he states. "I believe that the twenty-first century must be the century of human beings living in harmony with nature rather than being enslaved by technology."

Nature Is My God

The twentieth century has been one of the most tragic centuries, one with much bloodshed, domination, and destruction. It is the most paradoxical century. On the one hand, we have made big breakthroughs in knowledge, which have resulted in new technologies; on the other hand, because of these technological breakthroughs, such as nuclear weapons, our very survival is in jeopardy. We are witnessing a breakdown of the proper relationship between humankind and the rest of nature.

I believe that this situation has arisen because we have retreated from the perennial values. It is not that we need any new values; the most important thing is to try to revive the universally known values from which we have retreated.

As a young man, I took to heart the Communist ideals. A young soul certainly cannot reject things like justice and equality. These were the goals proclaimed by the Communists. But in reality that terrible Communist experiment brought about a repression of human dignity, while violence was used to impose that model on society. In the name of communism we abandoned basic human values. So when I came to power in the Soviet Union, I wanted to restore those values of openness and freedom. Whenever I had the chance,

I began to make changes. My philosophy is based on common sense, on a perception of measure and moderation. If, for example, freedom is not linked to morality, it is not freedom. It is permissiveness. It is just self-seeking rather than freedom.

Life has value in itself. Even if some methods are claimed to be progressive, if they result in destruction of life, they are unacceptable. I believe that the twenty-first century must be the century of human beings living in harmony with nature rather than being enslaved by technology.

We must encourage those who favor economic liberalism in Russia, but they must abandon the idea that they can use the ideological vacuum there to impose Westernization as a way to solve our problems. I think that economic liberalism is no less vulnerable than socialism or communism. Economic prosperity must go hand in hand with social cohesion and ecological sustainability. What good is a lot of money when the social fabric is destroyed and the environment polluted?

Values such as solidarity, a socially oriented economy, and the need to harmonize relations between humankind and the rest of nature are equally important. The future will depend on whether we will be able to find a synthesis, a fusion of ecological, liberal, and social values. These I call the perennial values.

I want to put great emphasis on the intrinsic value of nature, because without nature people cannot exist. We must preserve both people and nature. If we do not respect nature, we could eventually disappear; and once again on Earth we would have nature without humankind. Humans gaining better knowledge of themselves and their role in the cosmos is of paramount importance. If we do that, then we can ensure ourselves against many dangers. We should become more modest in terms of our needs and more respectful of the environment of which we are just a part.

If we do not learn to live in harmony with nature, we shall make our own lives hopeless, and we shall eventually jeopardize our own existence. In that sense I believe that we should go back to a new kind of renaissance based on people living more naturally.

We need to go back to the universal values in order to regain respect for our world. However difficult, we should try to preserve strategies that do not abandon those most important values. We should seek to incorporate those values in practical ways. First of all, we have to relinquish all kinds of violence. Second, we have to understand that we should not resort to extremism. Politicians in Russia, as elsewhere, need to understand that a free-market economy is no guarantee for safeguarding universal values. Once you have a free market, you will not find overnight that you are living in a free country. A lot of experience has to be gained in how to use freedom. So one has to be willing to go along the path step by step and incorporate other principles. If we fail to restore human dignity and ecological sustainability, the free market is of no use. If the social and the environmental costs of the free market are not taken into account, trust will evaporate. People today are disenchanted with politics. They do not trust politicians and feel that politicians regard them just as the means to power.

Without inspiration, all attempts at reform will fail. Human beings are not just dust in the air; they want to be involved in changing life for the better. Today, people with power in Russia are incapable of being in touch with the people who initially trusted them. The result is that the people have lost their inspiration; they live in a survival mode. This again cultivates the old mind-set, dependent on having a good tsar or general secretary. But in a country where many nations and ethnic groups live, you can only achieve your goals when the entire society is involved.

From my parents, I learned common sense, which is so typical of rural people. They have a feeling for nature, for the cosmos, for real life. They are born and live on the land. They have a feeling for that land. They raise their heads to the sky to see the clouds that bring rain and to look at the stars. People who are associated with the land interact with the stars. This association with nature gives people a very good hold on common sense.

I also learned modesty and humility. In rural communities there is a lot of very hard work that brings tolerance and solidarity, and this is something I saw in my family and in my village. This has remained with me throughout my life. I have never forgotten where I come from. Sometimes people whose roots are from peasant stock, whose families are barely literate, are embarrassed by it. But I am never embarrassed by it; in fact, I am proud of my rural roots.

I believe in the cosmos. All of us are linked to the cosmos. Look at the sun: if there is no sun, then we cannot exist. So nature is my god. To me, nature is sacred; trees are my temples and forests are my cathedrals.

I am not afraid of death; this does not mean I am indifferent to life. I like living. I am very curious and life is interesting. I am not a nihilist. I believe we come to the world and we will leave the world, but I do not think it will be without a trace. Death is not the end. Were I to know I was going to die, I would not make a big fuss about it. I would be living naturally as before. I would not want to use the remaining time to say anything special; I would use it to communicate and be in contact with nature. I remember when I went back to my village, wheat was growing. I saw a field of wheat, and in the evening I heard quails singing. It was like a symphony, a concert. Then, during the night, I saw all those stars in the sky, and I felt that I was being supported by nature and that I was dissolving into nature. So I would leave my remaining days for this kind of communication; I would not want to trouble the living with any message.

Love is a mystery of nature. It is good that it will always remain a mystery. Love for me is what unites two beings but it also unites humans and nature. I believe that we are dealing here with a mystery that is greater than us; once you try to define it, it is the end of love. It dies once you think you know the secret.

Will Keepin

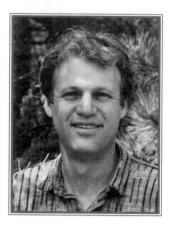

As an environmental scientist, Will Keepin was consultant physicist to the Energy Foundation. He now codirects the Shavano Institute in Colorado. Focusing on the important balance between social activism and listening to our hearts, he writes, "If we want a loving, compassionate world, then we must become loving and compassionate ourselves. . . . When we remake ourselves, then we remake the world, not the other way around."

Leading with Spirit

Transforming the Heart of Ecological Activism

I began my professional career in environmental science and technology, but over time it became clear to me that the roots of our ecological problems are neither technological nor scientific. Rather, the core of our ecological and social malaise is rooted in Western cultural values. My long-term goal has, therefore, shifted from transforming the industrial infrastructure to transforming the industrial mind-set, which entails a shift from promoting sustainable technologies in the heart of industry to implementing practices for transforming consciousness in the hearts of the citizens themselves.

In my early scientific work I specialized in energy research and worked at an institute in Austria doing research on global energy. The institute had developed a computer model of the world's energy future that called for covering the planet with nuclear power plants as the answer to our future energy needs. I soon learned that the zealous pro-nuclear research team was so married to a nuclear future that any critique of its technology or its computer forecast was interpreted as a personal attack or some kind of betrayal. I was stunned by the hubris and arrogance of this stance.

Over the next few years as I became engaged in alternative energy research—solar power, energy conservation, and so on—I slowly realized to my horror that I was becoming the same way, equally as inflexible and arrogant about the answers I had on solar energy as the nuclear advocates had been about their position. Moreover, I was constantly engaging in battle, becoming ever further encased around my position. This forced me into a deep personal inquiry that ultimately transformed my entire personal perspective and professional focus.

Out of that inquiry arose a vision of the future for ecological activism. I choose the term *vision* carefully, because vision has two fundamental meanings: an image of the future, such as a forecast of where things are going or perhaps ought to go, and the capacity to see. Though we often focus on the first definition, perhaps the second is ultimately more important. More than extraordinary visions of new realities, we need new eyes with which to see ordinary reality more clearly and the extraordinary opportunities before us.

There is currently a crisis in the ecology movement, an urgent need for new direction and fresh approaches. Part of the problem is that the environmental movement has tended to define itself by what it opposes: we're clear on what we are against, but we haven't developed an articulate vision of what we are for. We need to cultivate and develop our capacity for visioning, for this capacity is tragically devalued in our culture. The price of growing up in our society is giving up the vision or dream in our hearts, which we are taught to replace with the status quo reality. We are admonished not to hold any vision of the future that is unrealistic, but in that process we are robbed of both our cherished visions and our capacity to envision. So the first step in creating a future we want is to cultivate our powers of vision and to empower these visions with our hearts' yearning.

Another part of the problem is that we believe we must have a detailed blueprint before we can embark on building our dreams. But there are no maps and charts to get there. Our vision of the future is not something we know how achieve in advance; it's something we manifest over time by maintaining a deep conviction and taking one step at a time, correcting our course as we go. By our holding a vision deeply enough, it will become manifest; we bring into reality that which we hold in our imaginations. If we constantly hold the impossibility of a sustainable future, even unconsciously, we will definitely live into a future that is not sustainable. But if we begin to articulate the vision of a sustainable and desirable future and we hold this strongly in our hearts, we are synchronizing forces on many levels that will converge to bring this vision of the future into existence.

What is essential to revitalizing ecological activism is to bring the inner work of the heart into the outer work of service. Gandhi said, "Be the change that you want to see in the world!" That simple instruction has profound implications. If we want a loving, compassionate world, then we must become loving and compassionate ourselves, and that requires very specific tasks and practices. We can do this without any fanfare, without any kind of pretenses. We begin to be the change we want to see in the world, and thus we remake ourselves. When we remake ourselves, then we remake the world, not the other way around.

Martin Luther King, Jr., successfully applied Gandhi's spiritual principles in one of the most challenging cultural contexts imaginable. He identified four stages of direct spiritual action. The first is to compile the data that demonstrate the existence of an injustice. The second is to negotiate with the perpetrators, the authorities, or whoever is responsible for the injustice. The third is what King called purification, which is essentially doing the inner work of the heart. The fourth is direct action. It's a very simple program, and yet our dominant models of social change typically ignore or leave out the third step. We gather the data, we negotiate, and as soon as we don't get what we want, we go to court or to war. We move into action from a foundation of anger, frustration, or despair. What King calls purification we might in a more contemporary context call the inner work of the heart, the requisite personal and collective transformation that transforms the negative energies and motivations underlying our activism. In this way we become far more effective and compassionate agents for social change.

In the course of our work with social change advocates and ecological activists, especially those who are striving to integrate spiritual practice into their leadership and activism, we have developed a set of principles of spiritual leadership. These principles are certainly not definitive; rather they are an inquiry into how we can apply spiritual teachings to social-change work.

The first principle is that the motivation underlying our activism must be transformed from anger and despair to compassion and love. This is not to deny the legitimacy of noble anger or outrage at injustice of any kind. Rather, we seek to work for love instead of against evil. Even if our outer actions are the same, there is a major difference in results if our underlying intention is supporting love rather than defeating evil.

The second principle is a classical spiritual tenet, the principle of nonattachment to outcome. If our work is to foster lasting positive change, we must commit to doing something even if we never see the results in our own lifetime. This requires a deepening of faith in the intrinsic value of our work, beyond the concrete results. There is an old story about a great forest fire. All the animals run out of the forest and jump across the river to escape the fire, where they watch the fire consume their forest. They see a small bird swooping down and scooping up a drop of water in its beak from the river, then flying over the burning forest and releasing the drop of water onto the fire. The bird returns to the river for another drop and continues to release droplets of water onto the fire one at a time. Seeing this, the animals burst out laughing at the bird. "Why are you doing this? Your few pitiful drops are no match for this forest fire!" The bird replies, "I do it because it is what must be done." Then, of course, Providence takes notice of the purity of intent in this small bird and is so moved it creates a thunderstorm that puts out the fire.

In one of our workshops, there was a government lawyer from Washington, D.C., a powerful, heavy-hitting environmentalist. He reacted strongly to this principle and asked, "How can I possibly go into court and not be attached to the outcome? You bet I care who wins and who loses! If I am not attached to the outcome, I'll just get bulldozed!" His words illustrated the poignant challenge of implementing these principles in practice. Yet he keeps coming back to our retreats, actively seeking ways to love his adversaries. Once he acknowledged that although it was very difficult to love some of the unscrupulous people he has to deal with, he could at least love them for creating the opportunity for him to become a strong voice for truth and protection of the natural environment.

The third principle is that your integrity is your protection. If your work has integrity, then that itself will protect you. The fourth principle is related: the need for unified integrity in both means and ends. Integrity in means cultivates integrity in the fruit of our work; we cannot achieve a noble goal using ignoble means.

The fifth principle is not to demonize our adversaries. People respond to arrogance with their own arrogance, which leads to polarization. The ideal is to constantly entertain alternative points of view so that we move from arrogance to inquiry. Going into an adversarial situation, we can be aware of the correctness of what we are affirming, but there is usually a kernel of correctness, however small, of what is being affirmed by our opponent.

The sixth principle is to move from an "us-them" consciousness to a "we" consciousness. This means recognizing that we are the logger: when I write these principles of spiritual activism and publish them in this book, I am giving the command to the logger to fell the trees, to produce the pulp, to produce this paper so that I can publish these spiritual principles of activism about how best to save the trees. It is seeing the full circle of our interconnected complicity. We are not exempt and we are not different. The "them" that we talk about is also us.

The seventh principle is that our work is for the world rather than for us. We serve on behalf of others and not for our own satisfaction or benefit. We're sowing seeds for a cherished vision to become a future reality, and our fulfillment comes from the privilege of being able to do this work. This is the traditional understanding of selfless service. But then the eighth principle is that selfless service is a myth, because in serving others, we also serve ourselves. In giving, we receive. This is important to recognize so we don't fall into the trap of pretentious service to others' needs and develop a false sense of selflessness.

The ninth principle is not to insulate ourselves from the pain of the world. We must allow our hearts to be broken open. As we let that pain in, we become a vehicle for its transformation; if we block the pain, we prevent our own participation in the world's attempt to heal itself.

The tenth principle is what we attend to, we become. If we constantly attend to battles, we become embattled. On the other hand, if we constantly give love, we become loving. What we choose shapes and deeply defines us.

The eleventh principle is to rely on faith, defined here not as blind adherence to any set of beliefs but as a knowing from experience the universal principles beyond our direct observation. It is the responsibility of each of us to connect with what our unique role is, while trusting that the rest will work itself out.

Finally, the twelfth principle is that love creates the form. It is the mind that gives rise to the apparent fragmentation of the world, while the heart operates at greater depth. When we bring the fullness of our humanity to our activism, we can be far more effective in creating the future we envision.

As we enter the third millennium, we are urgently called to action in two distinct capacities: to serve as hospice workers to a dying culture and to serve as midwives to an emerging culture. We must cultivate the requisite compassion to skillfully bear the grief and loss associated with the passing of the material and ecological excesses of twentieth-century society, while bringing into existence a new culture, which requires new forms of organization and ecological communities and unprecedented forms of harmony between diverse peoples. These two tasks are required simultaneously. The key is to root our actions in both intelligence and compassion—a balance of head and heart that combines the finest human qualities—in our leadership for cultural transformation.

Thich Nhat Hanh

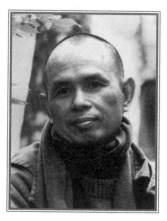

Vietnamese Zen master, poet, and peace activist, Thich Nhat Hanh is a prolific writer and beloved teacher. In his piece he focuses on the path of harmlessness, or ahimsa. "If we divide reality into two camps—the violent and the nonviolent—and stand in one camp while attacking the other, the world will never have peace."

Ahimsa

The Path of Environmental Interbeing

The Sanskrit word *ahimsa,* usually translated as nonviolence, literally means nonharming or harmlessness. To practice ahimsa, we first have to practice it within ourselves. In each of us, there is both a certain amount of violence and a certain amount of nonviolence. Depending on our state of being, our response to things is more or less nonviolent. But even if we take pride in being vegetarian, for example, we have to acknowledge that the water in which we boil our vegetables contains many tiny microorganisms. We cannot be completely nonviolent, but we can go in the direction of nonviolence. If we want to head north, we can use the North Star to guide us. It is impossible to arrive at the North Star, but our effort is to proceed in that direction.

If we divide reality into two camps—the violent and the nonviolent—and stand in one camp while attacking the other, the world will never have peace. We will always blame and condemn those we feel are responsible for wars and social injustice, without recognizing the degree of violence in ourselves. We must work on ourselves as well as with those we condemn if we wish to move toward peace. It never helps to draw a line and dismiss some people as enemies, even those who act violently. We have to approach them with love in our hearts and do our best to help them move in a direction of nonviolence. If we work for peace out of anger, we will never succeed. Peace can never come about through nonpeaceful means.

If we look deeply, we can observe that the roots of war are in the unmindful ways we have been living. We have not sown enough seeds of peace and understanding in ourselves and others; therefore we are co-responsible: because I have been like this, they are like that. With this insight, we can see clearly. Then we can go to a demonstration and say, "This war is unjust, destructive, and not worthy of our great nation." This is far more effective than angrily condemning others. Anger always accelerates the damage.

All of us, even pacifists, have pain inside. We feel angry and frustrated, and we need to find someone willing to listen to us who is capable of understanding our suffering. In Buddhist iconography, there is a bodhisattva named Avalokitesvara who has one thousand arms and one thousand hands, with an eye in the palm of each hand. The one thousand hands represent action, and the one thousand eyes represent understanding. When you understand a situation or a person, any action you take will help and will not cause more suffering. When you have an eye in your hand, you will know how to practice nonviolence.

Imagine if each of our words also had an eye in it. Before we said something, we would have to understand what we were saying and the person to whom our words were directed. With the eye of understanding, we would not say things to make the other person suffer. Blaming and arguing are forms of violence. If we are suffering, then when we speak, our words may be bitter and not help anyone. We have to learn to calm ourselves before we speak. This is the art of loving speech.

Listening is also a loving practice. Avalokitesvara has a great talent for listening; in Chinese, his name means "listening to the cries of the world." We have to listen so that we understand the suffering of others; we have to empty ourselves and leave space so we can listen well. Just by listening deeply, we can alleviate a great deal of pain. This is an important practice of peace. We have to listen in our families and in our communities. We have to listen to everyone, especially those we consider our enemies. When we show our capacity for listening and understanding, the other person will also listen to us, and we will have a chance to speak of our pain. This is the beginning of healing.

Thinking is at the base of everything, so it is important for us to put an eye of awareness into each of our thoughts. Without a correct understanding of a situation or a person, our thoughts can be misleading and create confusion, despair, anger, or hatred. Our most important task is to develop correct insight. If we see deeply into the nature of interbeing, we will stop blaming, arguing, and killing, and we will become friends with everyone.

These are the three domains of action: body, speech, and mind. There is also nonaction, which is often more important than action. If we want to help the world, the practice of nonviolent nonaction is often essential; things can sometimes go more smoothly without our doing anything, just because of our peaceful presence. We can practice nonaction in the domain of speech: words can create understanding, but they can also cause others to suffer. Sometimes it is best not to say anything.

We can practice ahimsa in our world. Although we human beings are animals, a part of nature, we single ourselves out from nature, thinking of other animals and living beings as nature and acting as if we are not a part of it. Then we ask, "How should we deal with nature?" The answer is we should deal with it the way we should deal with ourselves. Just as we should not harm ourselves, we should not harm nature. In fact, to harm nature is to harm ourselves.

We humans think we are smart, but an orchid, for example, knows how to produce noble, symmetrical flowers, and a snail knows how to make a beautiful, well-proportioned shell. Compared with their knowledge, ours is not worth much at all. We should bow deeply before the orchid and the snail and join our palms reverently before the monarch butterfly and the magnolia tree. The feeling of respect for all species will help us recognize the noblest nature in ourselves.

If you are a mountain climber or someone who enjoys the countryside or the forest, you know that forests are our lungs outside of our bodies. Yet we have been acting in a way that has allowed two million square miles of land to be deforested. At the same time we have created acid rain and destroyed the rivers and parts of the ozone layer. We are each imprisoned in our small self, thinking only of some more comfort for this small self, while we destroy our large self. If we want to change the situation, we must begin by being the forest, the river, and the ozone layer. If we visualize ourselves as the forest, we will experience the hopes and fears of the trees. When we understand that we inter-are with the trees, we know that if they do not live, we too will disappear and that it is up to us to make an effort to keep the trees alive.

Everything is in transformation. All life is impermanent. We are all children of the earth, and, at some time, she will take us back to her again. We are continually arising from Mother Earth, being nurtured by her, and then returning to the earth. Like us, plants are born, live for a while, and then return to the earth. When they decompose, they fertilize our gardens. Living vegetables and decomposing vegetables are part of the same reality. Without one, the other cannot be.

Plants and the earth rely on each other, as they also rely on us. Our way of walking on the earth has a great influence on animals and plants. We have killed many animals and plants and destroyed their environment. In turn, our environment is now harming us. Polluted water and air are taking their toll. We are like sleepwalkers, not knowing what we are doing or where we are heading. Whether we can wake up depends on whether we can walk mindfully on our Mother Earth. The future of all life, including our own, depends on our mindful steps.

So many beings in the universe love us unconditionally. The trees, the water, and the air do not ask anything of us; they just love us. Even though we need this kind of love, we continue to destroy them. By destroying the animals, the air, and the trees, we are destroying ourselves. Our ecology should be a universal ecology. If the earth were our body, we would be able to feel many areas where she is suffering. We must learn to practice unconditional love for all beings so that the animals, the air, and the trees can continue to be themselves. If we can change our daily lives—the way we think, the way we speak, the way we act—we can change the world.

So to practice ahimsa, we must learn ways to deal peacefully with ourselves; we must become ahimsa, so that when a situation presents itself, we will not create more suffering. We need gentleness, loving-kindness, compassion, joy, and equanimity directed to our bodies, our feelings, other people, and our environment. Peace must be based on insight and understanding, and for this we must practice deep reflection—looking into each act and each thought of our daily lives.

Mindfulness enables us to do this by helping us be fully present in each moment. We normally spend so much time worrying about the future or regretting the past, and we get carried away by our thinking. Overwhelmed by our sorrows and anxieties, we need to cultivate the energy of mindfulness to come back to the present and to encounter life in this moment. The only moment for us to be truly alive is the present moment. To be present, we breathe in deeply, aware of the fact that we are alive, and as we breathe out, we smile to life. If we breathe in and out consciously like this, just three times, our body and mind will come together. Usually our mind is in one place—in the past or the future—and our body is somewhere else. After we breathe in and out consciously, we find that we are really here, in this moment.

It is in this moment that we can prevent war or the next crisis. When a crisis has begun, it is already too late. If we and our children practice ahimsa in our daily lives and if we learn how to plant seeds of peace and reconciliation in our own hearts and minds, we will begin to establish peace. How much time does it take to breathe consciously, to smile, and to be fully present in each moment? Our real enemy is forgetfulness. If we nourish mindfulness every day and water the seeds of peace in ourselves and those around us, we have a good chance to prevent the next war and to defuse the next crisis.

The seeds of joy and freedom are buried deep in our consciousness. If we do not water these seeds, peace will never be obtained. We run away from ourselves because we do not want to touch our pain, suffering, anger, or despair. In today's society, everything encourages us to run away from ourselves and look outside for happiness. So it is important for us to learn to embrace our pain, anger, and fear in a very tender way, to accept them, and to make our peace with them. The energy of mindfulness will help us. When we do this, a transformation takes place and we touch the deep peace, joy, and stability that are within us.

Hanne Strong

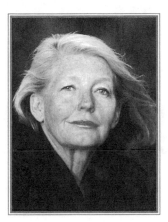

H̃anne Strong has established the Earth Restoration Corps (ERC), an educational program for young adults to learn essential skills in respecting, restoring, and caring for Earth. Sharing her vision of the ERC, she says, "The point is to provide the next generation with the tools to restore Earth and themselves. . . . The security of humanity will not require armies of soldiers but battalions of conscious environmentalists."

A Conscious Revolution of Conscience

These are critical times. In critical times, it is of utmost importance to realistically assess the situation in a very direct, practical way. It does not matter what philosophy we hold or what religion we follow; we cannot avoid the reality of the condition of our environment, our social systems, and our personal consciousness. The crisis is as immediate as the earth we stand on, the air we breathe, the water we drink, and the sun we live beneath.

The basis for cooperative human relations and environmental awareness is a moral and spiritual core. We have lost touch with this. Our root problem, from which the crisis has arisen, is that we are living out of balance with ourselves, each other, and our Earth. If we do not take steps to see how the destruction of the environment is an outward reflection of the imbalance within ourselves, then the environment will continue to show it to us in ever more dramatic ways. Our present solutions to environmental and interpersonal problems are only Band-Aids. If we want our external world to change, we must change first within ourselves.

To begin with, we need to become aware of our inherent connection to the earth and embrace the importance of living by the natural law. This includes the law of cause and effect and the law of interdependence. It is a simple matter to observe the correlation between cause and effect: if we are greedy, we do not hesitate to exploit the earth; if we are peaceful, we will not create chaos. Our internal environment—our minds—and our external environment—the world—are intimately interrelated. In ignoring the law of cause and effect, we fail to understand the results of our actions. We look outside ourselves for answers, instead of living and acting for the benefit of the whole, which is the law of interdependence.

Nature consists of four elements—water, earth, fire, and air. The interdependence between all living beings and these vital elements creates either balance or imbalance. Presently, we choose to discount a basic natural law, which is, "Never take more than you need and always give something back." We take excessively from the earth and return these gifts with poison and garbage. Where is our gratitude and respect? We are receiving our medicines, our food, our very existence from Earth, yet we waste water, pollute the air, poison the soil, raze the forests, and destroy our protection from the sun.

If we are to survive, we must raise our sights toward supporting the immediate development of the highest aspect of being human within ourselves and help to inspire others to participate. It is time to move away from the need for money, power, and materialism. During these critical times we must recognize our obligation to provide the next generation with a new direction and vision.

At the Earth Summit in Rio de Janeiro in 1992, world leaders asked whether modern society is sustainable on the planet without fundamental change. The answer is no. What, then, is the fundamental change that must take place if the human race is to survive?

What is called for is a conscious revolution of the conscience. As there is so little time available, a revolution is necessary. This is a very different revolution from uprisings of the past. This revolution is to save the Earth and ourselves from destruction. I suggest that we need a strategy similar to the Marshall Plan in which we, as a world community, unify our efforts to restore the spirit of humanity and of the earth. I am calling this a conscious revolution of the conscience. As conscious revolutionaries we need to focus on two key problems affecting us: environmental destruction and the loss of the next generation. These two are directly linked. The meeting point is to provide the next generation with the tools to restore the earth and themselves by offering ways to explore the meaning of being a human on this planet. We can teach the next generation that there are alternative solutions to the endless cycle of working for low wages and spending money on objects that deplete our natural resources.

Many youth of today can see the destructiveness and meaninglessness of the actions of our generation. They reflect this by living bored, selfish, violent, addictive, self-destructive lives. The young especially are in great need of discovering purpose and dignity in their lives. The question is how to capture their enthusiasm and motivate them before they become mired in further self-destruction. They are in need of guidance, inspired vision, and the right tools to make the changes we are so unable to make ourselves.

For past generations, the transition from youth to adulthood meant getting a driver's license and credit cards and gleefully moving into a materialistic world. We have paid a great price for this in terms of our future. We must not seduce the next generation into following our example.

Many alternatives for such a transition into adulthood are based on practices in the traditional cultures in which the elders take young people into nature to learn the basic tenets of the earth and the cosmos. They learn what it means to become an inherently viable participant in preserving and honoring all life. The emerging adults are asked to seek their vision and life plan in terms of their place within their society; they are given the tools to develop a conscience centered in a basic understanding and reverence for the earth. The impact of spending time in nature, unprotected by modern conveniences and therefore vulnerable to the elements, while surrounded by the sacredness and grandness of nature, has a great influence on any human being. Nature can be merciless as well as nurturing, confronting as well as embracing.

In light of this, one solution I propose is the establishment of an Earth Restoration Corps (ERC). This is a training program, held in Crestone, Colorado, designed to encourage and support the transformation of individual perceptions and values within a context of learning sustainable ways and techniques in balance with nature. From this training the participants are encouraged to assume the leadership necessary for remedial action on behalf of the earth. It instills ethical and spiritual integrity as a basis for cooperative human relations and environmentally responsible living.

An experience in nature, such as the ERC program, stimulates the capacity to handle unforeseen circumstances and unpredictable events in alignment with intent and generosity of spirit. Often these events spark moments of transcendence and inspired creative action. The training makes use of both modern science and traditional wisdom, bridging the best of current sustainable technologies with the best of indigenous wisdom. This provides the conditions for participants to learn to care deeply and skillfully for Earth and for one another.

The ERC participant lives in a wilderness environment and spends time alone on a solo experience. It is out of this experience that the understanding of morality, respect, love, and wisdom takes on a true meaning in everyday life. Each participant begins to consciously develop a personal value system within an environmentally sensitive context.

In addition, participants are taught skills in leadership; conflict resolution; sustainable building, farming, and gardening techniques; land, water, forest, air, and soil restoration; renewable energy source handling; water management; and preventive health care. During previous programs, we have had participants from the Philippines, Bhutan, Australia, Russia, Spain, Central and South America, and Africa. Many of the ERC trainees arrive from a city and have had no experience of nature prior to this training. By the end of six weeks, the participants have the training to return to their homelands to continue the ERC program, to initiate and facilitate community projects, to seek employment in sustainable development fields, and to live in an environmentally sensitive manner.

On the basis of employment projections, two billion youths, especially from third world countries, will enter the world's job market in the next few years. To accomplish our goal of providing jobs for our youth, massive training programs based on the ERC program are needed worldwide.

The ERC leadership training program is the beginning of the conscious revolution of the conscience. As each participant returns to his or her homeland, the global community will begin to feel the impact. The seeds of this knowledge have the potential to sprout into meaningful jobs, national service systems, and prison reform programs. The present six-week intensive program needs to be expanded into a two-year program. It needs to be a national service system that every country puts in place. The armed services of each country can use the ERC leadership training as a basis to provide alternative service for young adults who wish to defend the earth as well as their country. The money used to train fighters could be redirected to train in the skills necessary for our future. The security of humanity, as well as our survival, will not require armies of soldiers but battalions of conscious environmentalists. Our security depends on a healthy environment.

In the future, just imagine every country has a two-year national service program in which the youth learn how to restore Earth and develop personal ethics. Just visualize governments redirecting the billions spent on incarcerating rebellious youths toward retraining them to live ecologically responsible and humanly sensitive lives. This is what I dream for the world's future.

The stakes have never been higher, nor the choices more compelling. Overwhelming evidence indicates that humanity's present direction is leading to an irrevocable loss of the natural systems that support all life as we know it, a severely diminished existence, and an unknown but clearly compromised future. It is the duty of every human being to develop the highest aspect of being human.

We must become conscious of our responsibility to each other and to the next generation. We have a lot of work to do to turn around our present destruction of the Earth to one of restoration. We can't just address the symptoms; we have to go to the root of the problem which is the human spirit. Unless that changes, nothing will. Only when we experience the interconnectedness of all life can we begin to change human consciousness and begin to live as enlightened caretakers of the Earth.

Kitaro

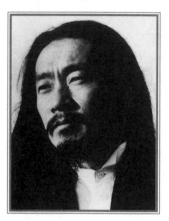

A renowned musician and poet, Kitaro has a singular style of contemporary music that has made him famous worldwide. The following contribution illustrates his belief in nature and the spirit of humankind.

Time and Life

Passage of time is of continuous moments
Life is undulation of moments and of
Continuous energy
Macro to micro
Micro to macro
From one dimension to another
It continuously transports
Sometimes slowly
Sometimes rapidly
As time goes by
It crosses over dimension to another
Nature and life crosses
Yin and yang crosses
Nature as it is
Life as it is
Far beyond the passage of time
And any dimensions
May life be eternal
May life be eternal
always

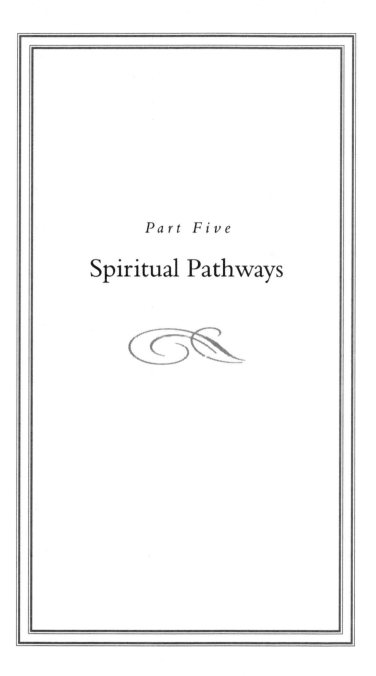

Part Five

Spiritual Pathways

Archbishop Desmond Tutu

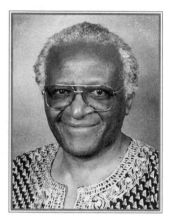

Recipient of the Nobel Peace Prize in 1984 and archbishop emeritus of South Africa, Archbishop Tutu is now leading the Commission for Truth and Reconciliation to bring to a conclusion some of the apartheid atrocities. In this piece he shares his passion for forgiveness, saying, "Without forgiveness human society and existence are impossible."

Becoming More Fully Human

I was born in a Christian family, so in a way my religious belief was given to me through my mother's milk. It felt very natural—a process unfolding—I was doing what came naturally to me without having to think about it. I went for training as a priest because the government introduced education for black people, but it was very inferior education. I refused to be a collaborator in this travesty of an education. There were very few options, so I went to a theological seminary. I opposed apartheid and all its actions that leave so many homeless or destroyed because it so completely contradicts my faith. I was opposed to apartheid not out of political conviction but because I was a Christian.

During the struggle it was exhilarating to be upheld and supported by the love and prayers from so many around the world. Our victory would have been totally impossible without that support of our sisters and brothers. Now we are trying to deal with our past, to heal the wounds apartheid inflicted, to pour balm on them, and to reconcile a traumatized and wounded people.

When someone is in pain or suffering, we need to sit with that person and seek to enter into her or his pain and agony. Then we can speak with some credibility out of that shared solidarity. If we do not share and enter into pain together, it is like praising fasting when your own stomach is full.

Without forgiveness human society and existence are impossible. We are forever hurting one another, forever stepping on one another's toes. So we have to forgive and be forgiven or else we cannot go on living full lives. To forgive is not to pretend that the wrong is not awful and hurtful. It is to accept it in all its awfulness and pain and to want to give the other person the chance to begin again.

We learn how to forgive by forgiving, but we can't teach people how to forgive. We can only hope that they will imitate those who do forgive. Jesus taught by example as we saw Him being nailed on the cross and praying for his tormentors. "Father, forgive them, for they do not know what they are doing" moves us to emulate Him.

I draw my strength from prayer. Without prayer, life for me would be impossible. When I have not prayed, what I feel is almost physical, like not brushing my teeth. Prayer is totally indispensable to put me in touch with the Transcendent, the Omnipotent, the Source of all life, love, and goodness. I depend, too, on the prayers of others because I belong in a family—the human family, God's family. It is clear, therefore, that I try to let my praying fill my entire life; my life is a working out of my praying.

My encounter with God has repercussions for my life with my neighbor, for how can I love God, whom I have not seen, if I hate my neighbor, whom I have seen? My God is one who says, "In as much as you have done it to the least of these, my brothers and sisters, you have done it to me."

I want to see a world that would be as God intended it to be—more gentle, more caring, more compassionate, in which people mattered more than things, more than profits, in which children could play and not learn how to hate, not be used as child soldiers taught to kill when they should be playing, in which we would not spend such obscene amounts on budgets of death and destruction but would ensure that children have decent homes, adequate education and health care, clean water, and a safe environment.

We should all become instruments of peace, love, and compassion, and so impregnate the atmosphere with these, rather than with their ghastly counterparts. You know when you enter a happy home. You don't have to be told; you don't have to see the happy people who live there. You can feel it in the fabric, the air. You know when you enter a church that is prayed in; you sense the prayerfulness, the reverence, the holiness in the very stones. So we too can ensure that the ether, the air we breathe, is packed chockablock with goodness, truth, love, laughter, joy, caring, and compassion!

We should help people to become more fully human so that we can celebrate our diversity, celebrate who we are in our various languages, cultures, religions, traditions, and give others space to be what God wants them to be, uniquely themselves. So we should inspire in all the spirit of tolerance, a deep reverence for human life and for beauty and goodness.

You are a V.S.P.—a Very Special Person. You are God's viceroy, God's representative. You are God's stand-in, a God carrier. You are precious; God depends on you. God believes in you and has no one but you to do the things that only you can do for God. Become what you are.

Sri Swami Satchidananda

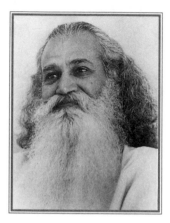

From India to Sri Lanka to the United States, Swamiji is loved by many as a messenger of peace. The founder of Integral Yoga institutes, which bring the yogic path to students worldwide, he focuses on the spiritual path and the need for us to find the teacher within ourselves. "When we hear the inner teacher," he says, "it will say something for the benefit or sake of everybody, while the ego will always say something for our own sake."

The Inner Guru

The world is about to go through an awakening. Before an awakening there is a dark cloud; just before the dawn it is the darkest. We are in a chaotic place, but that is the sign that people are about to awaken, that real change is coming, that we will create a better world. This is the darkest stage right now, so the next stage is the dawn. Our time is different from cosmic time, so however long it takes, heaven will wait. Children have a game that is an obstacle race. They put a lot of obstacles in the way, and you have to go through them—under the carpet and through the barrel and over the wall. Well, suppose somebody avoids all that and goes around the obstacles and then asks for the winner's cup. Will they give him or her the cup? No, the person has to prove he or she is capable of going through the obstacles. In the same way, we are having to face the obstacles confronting all humans.

When you see the darkness not as darkness but as a part of the day, then you know that there is always light and darkness. So when you see the dark, you know the light will come. The one who sees both ups and downs, profit and loss, praise and blame, pain and sorrow as equal is like a good surfer. Some people don't know how to surf and so they get caught in the waves; in surfing you have to move with the waves. Good surfers don't get affected by the ups and downs as they keep their minds above the waves of the ocean. Similarly, sorrow and pleasure, pain and joy, profit and loss, all make one complete circle, just as both a depression and a crest make a wave.

There are many roles we can play in this life. When you put on a costume and play the drama, you do all kinds of things, but are you really doing it? Suppose in the play you are a male putting on a female act. You may play the role but you don't become female. On the stage, when you cry, are you really crying? If you don't really cry, people in the audience will laugh at you. So for the people it should appear that you are really crying, but within yourself do you cry? A person with wisdom will do everything like everybody else but she or he will not be affected by it. For the sake of the drama she or he does things, not for personal satisfaction or pleasure. She or he is doing it to play the part.

When I sit in a big chair and you sit in a smaller one, I am playing my part and you are playing your part. That doesn't mean I'm big and you are small. Essentially we are the same, but we are playing different roles in life. It is fun to do this, as long as we remember we are essentially all equal. I'm just playing my part, but at the same time I should not forget myself. And if I know myself, I should know yourself too, for in that self we are all equal. That is what we call spiritual understanding. The different roles make us different but in spirit we are one. If we have that spiritual vision, we aren't affected by anything. God doesn't differentiate between Saddam Hussein and Bill Clinton. It's Saddam Hussein and Bill Clinton who think that they are Hussein or Clinton. But to God there is no difference; they are both His people.

There is difference and there is oneness. We are all one in spirit but many in minds and bodies. Our bodies are different, our minds are different, our thinking is different. We are different in hundreds of ways. But at the same time we are one in spirit. Realize that one-ness. Gold is one, yet how many varieties of ornaments do we make? How many names do we give them—rings, chains, or bangles—yet whatever the names they are still just gold. So there is oneness and manyness.

Go to the sea and what do we see? Waves, icebergs, foam, bub-bles, spray—they all have their own names. Yet is the wave different from water? Is the spray different from water? Is the iceberg different from water? Because they appear different, we use different names. Take, for example, the chess game. What do we have on the board? King, queen, bishop, and so on. We call the pieces these names, but they're all chipped off the same block; they are all wood or marble. As soon as we put them on the board, they have separateness; they have their own movements. This means we are one in essence but many in nonsense!

Keep good company. Whatever you want to achieve, you have to have the right company. If you want to enjoy drinking, you can't have the company of yogis; you have to have the company of drinkers. Whatever you want to experience, you should have the company that will be conducive to that experience. Practice medita-tion and watch your thoughts. Practice loving service. Do the right thing for the sake of others. That way, slowly, the mind becomes clean, becomes balanced. In the Bible one of the beatitudes is "Blessed are the sufferers." How can that holy book say suffering people are blessed people? Because suffering is the only way to clean something. Suppose the linen gets dirty. What do you do? You wash it, clean it out. Through suffering, the linen gets clean. Without suf-fering, it won't be clean.

My mission is to serve. Whenever the opportunity comes, I am here to serve. Everybody is created for that purpose. Animals, trees, plants, rain, and sun—they are not here for their own sake. They are being more useful to everybody else than to themselves. Only human beings think of themselves first. A tree brings forth many fruits, but it does not eat even one fruit. It gives all the fruit away. So we learn a lesson from the tree: to live for the sake of others rather than for ourselves.

You may want to serve but you must start with a clean instrument. When you want to perform an operation, the first thing you do is sterilize the instruments. Only then can you operate. Service is doing something, so it is like an operation. But you cannot serve well with a dirty mind or with selfish reasons, so you must serve yourself before you serve others. You prepare yourself. For instance, you may need to find the cause for your feelings, like anger. Perhaps you expect something to happen, and when it doesn't, you are angry. In this case, nobody brought you anger; you created your anger yourself. And your anger may not hurt anybody else, but it has already affected you, already created an unhealthy reaction in your body and mind.

Don't be angry. If you need to show your anger, show it. But don't become anger. If you become anger, in what way are you better than anyone else, better than a dictator, a terrorist, or even a rapist? Even if someone did something terrible to you, he or she did it with ignorance and foolishness, not with awareness. You don't have to be angry; pray for that person. Forgive. If you are keeping anger within you, it is going to affect your whole life. Keep good things, but forgive and forget bad things.

The guru, or teacher, is within you; your own mind is a teacher. Your guru does not have to be outside as a separate person. The duty of the outer guru is simply to show you the inner guru. When we hear the inner teacher, it will say something for the benefit or sake of everybody, while the ego will always say something for our own sake. So, in a way, the selfless ego is God, while the selfish god is ego.

This world is a university. Everybody is our teacher; we are only the students. We can learn from everything, not just people. The fan goes round and round. Does it revolve for its own sake or to give us cool air? Its nature is to revolve. A candle gives light. The candle doesn't know it is giving light; its nature is to give light. So the universe around us is, just by its nature, a great teacher. If we are willing to listen, to learn, and to serve, then we will be free.

Rick Fields

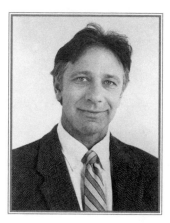

A poet, author, past editor of New Age Journal *and current editor of* Yoga Journal, *Rick Fields explores the mystery of our ultimate surrender.*

The Very Short Sutra on the Meeting
of the Buddha and the Goddess

Thus I have made up:
Once the Buddha was walking along the
forest path, walking without
arriving anywhere
or having any thought of arriving or not arriving
and lotuses shining with the morning dew
miraculously appeared under every step
soft as silk beneath the toes of the Buddha

When suddenly, out of the turquoise sky,
dancing in front of his half-shut inward-looking
eyes, shimmering like a rainbow
or a spider's web
transparent as the dew on a lotus flower
the Goddess appeared quivering
like a humming bird in the air before him.

She, for she was surely a she
as the Buddha could clearly see
with his eye of discriminating awareness wisdom,
was mostly red in colour

though when the light shifted
she flashed like a rainbow.

She was naked except
for the usual flower ornaments
Goddesses wear
Her long hair
was deep blue, her two eyes fathomless pits of space
and her third eye a bloodshot
ring of fire.

The Buddha folded his hands together
and greeted the Goddess thus:

"O Goddess, why are you blocking my path?
Before I saw you I was happily going nowhere.
Now I'm not sure where to go."

"You can go around me,"
said the Goddess, twirling on her heels like a bird
darting away,
but just a little way away,
"or you can come after me.
This is my forest too,
you can't pretend I'm not here."

With that the Buddha sat
    supple as a snake
    solid as a rock
beneath a Bo tree
    that sprang full-leaved
    to shade him.

"Perhaps we should have a chat,"
he said.
"After years of arduous practice
at the time of the morning star
I penetrated reality, and now . . ."

"Not so fast, Buddha.
I am reality."
The Earth stood still,
the oceans paused,
the wind itself listened
a thousand arhats, bodhisattvas and dakinis
magically appeared to hear
what would happen in the conversation.

"I know I take my life in my own hands,"
said the Buddha.
"But I am known as the Fearless One
so here goes."

And he and the Goddess
without further words
exchanged glances.

Light rays like sunbeams
shot forth
so bright that even
Sariputra, the All-Seeing One,
had to turn away.

And then they exchanged thoughts
and the illumination was as bright as a diamond candle.

And then they exchanged mind

And there was a great silence as vast as
the universe
that contains everything.

And then they exchanged bodies
and clothes

And the Buddha arose
as the Goddess
and the Goddess
arose as the Buddha

And so on back and forth
for a hundred thousand kalpas.

If you meet the Buddha
you meet the Goddess,
If you meet the Goddess
you meet the Buddha.

Not only that. This:
The Buddha is the Goddess,
the Goddess is the Buddha.

And not only that. This:
The Buddha is emptiness
the Goddess is bliss,
the Goddess is emptiness
the Buddha is bliss.

And that is what
and what–not you are
It's true.

So here comes the mantra of the Goddess and the Buddha, the un-
surpassed non-dual mantra. Just to say this mantra, just to hear this
mantra once, just to hear one word of this mantra once makes everything the way it truly is: OK.

So here it is:
    Earth-walker/sky-walker
        Hey, silent one, Hey, great talker
    Not two/not one
        Not separate/Not apart
    This is the heart
        Bliss is emptiness
        Emptiness is bliss
    Be your breath, Ah
    Smile, Hey
And relax, Ho
And remember this: You can't miss.

Ram Dass

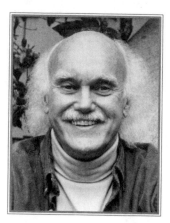

Venturing to India in the 1960s, Richard Alpert met his guru, Neem Karoli Baba, who renamed him Ram Dass. Returning to the West, he became a compassionate and forthright spiritual teacher. Here he explores the basis of spirituality, saying that "true compassionate action comes out of the awareness that we are all inseparable. . . . We are all part of the same thing, and therefore your suffering is my suffering."

On Hearing What Is

My involvement with the spiritual path evolved directly out of my experiences with teonanacatl, the "flesh of the gods" mushrooms, given to me by Tim Leary. There's no doubt that my initial experience was a spiritual one; for the first time, I acknowledged that there was a deeper part of my being, that I was more than just a body and a mind. Psychedelics (or entheogens, as I prefer to call them) opened me to different planes of consciousness, which in turn led me to focus on the nature of my own mind. I started to practice meditation, beginning with Vipassana and Hindu meditation, then Dzogchen and Tibetan Buddhism.

I think of meditation as a base camp for almost all my other spiritual practices because it has brought a deeply reflective quality into my life. It has changed my ability to hear and to function in many respects. I certainly see the difference if I don't meditate! I lose my foundation very easily; I get off center, get trapped in my desires or my fears, or go around with a lot of ill-digested experiences coloring my life. I get caught in my ego, in being righteous, in being an achiever, in being loved, in being important, in being helpful; I get caught in being something. It starts the journey of stress—of more is better and all of that. Every time I get lost in ego, there is stress. And then I come back to my meditative mindfulness, to my quiet presence, to my soul, and I see the dance of ego for what it is. When I sit and quiet down, I clean out my system and get back to center and emptiness, to joy and delight, and then I start to play again in the world.

Meditation leads us to see ego from a new perspective. The way I'm working with the concept of ego is by reducing all the different planes of consciousness to just three: ego, soul, and awareness. I use the term *ego* to refer to the cognitive map that describes who we are and how we organize all our sense and thought material. It's our conceptual map of reality; it's our software for functioning on this plane. It is who we think we are. And because it is taught to us by other people, our ego is rooted in our relationships.

But then there comes an awakening to a spiritual identity, one in which we are still a separate and unique identity—a soul—but in which we are much closer to God, much closer to the One. I see soul as a universal wisdom—as a central presence but one that is still identified with uniqueness. The soul is a set of factors forcing manifestation. The soul has karma, and part of its karma is that it manifests in this incarnation, but it's basically just using this incarnation to work out its karma.

Most of our spiritual work has to do with extricating ourselves from ego and moving to soul—going from an identification with our thoughts, with our conceptual map, to the cultivation of the witness, of a mindfulness or metaspace in which the whole game of incarnation and ego is being appreciated like a play or a dance. And then, as we get more established in that soul, the deeper yearning to come back into pure, undifferentiated awareness becomes stronger. That's the source of the poetry of Rumi or Kabir, the poetry of the Beloved. Bhakti, or devotion, is the yearning of the soul to be one with God.

The soul wants to want to be one with God—but not quite yet!

We're not sure we are quite ready to give up the deliciousness of the foreplay into the ecstasy of the orgasm. The funny thing is, when we finally surrender our separateness in order to merge with the Beloved, we find that in the merging we are also separate; so we get to have our cake and eat it too! All we have lost is the supremacy of the illusion of our separateness. Once there is just awareness, awareness is; it includes trees and rivers and us and everything. It is no longer "us," it is just awareness.

Now we can have that experience; we can enter into that space and still come back into the ego. In fact, that happens thousands and thousands of times. The soul tastes awareness for a moment, and then gets catapulted back. And that goes on for as long as the soul has karma. The clinging to any attraction or aversion keeps creating forms—incarnations or dream states—in which we keep working the stuff out.

Drawing back from identification with the ego does not mean that the ego stops functioning. It just means we are no longer functioning it, just as with our heart: our heart is beating; we are not beating it. In the same way, the ego goes on working, keeping the game together; we are just not busy doing it anymore. And the soul goes on too, because it's still running off old karma, only now there is nobody in there to create new karma. We are free, because awareness is free, God is free.

Yet the ego level is always at work. Take anger, for instance. I still get angry. The difference is that now I try to give it up as fast as I can. That's what my guru told me to do. He said, "Ram Dass, give up anger!" That was good advice, because anger is not a good strategy. It comes out of ego, out of righteousness. Anger comes from holding a model of how you think the world ought to be but isn't.

The aim of martial arts, which attempt to act out of a place of stillness, is to absolutely empty ourselves of intent, to sit in the center and experience the whole universe, so as to figure out the appropriate action. Anger thwarts that process of emptying and centering. It polarizes us into "for" and "against," and so creates separation. We have to cultivate compassion.

Anger arises out of judgment, and the judging mind is tricky to work with. I try to substitute appreciation for judgment whenever I can. If I go out into the woods, and I see trees of different shapes and sizes and colors, I admire and appreciate them without judging them, without saying, "An oak is better than an elm." But somehow, with humans, it's a whole other ball game; our egos get more involved.

A lot of our anger springs from the way our egos hold onto the past. It's so important to keep bringing ourselves into the present moment, in which the past has a part to play but does not dominate the scene. Then our identity is no longer with the past, with all the historical labels we've attached to ourselves, but with the present. Who did what to whom is all just mind stuff.

In the various Eastern traditions they say that life is a dream. It's like falling asleep and dreaming. Or it's like changing channels on the television set: what was on channel 5 is no longer there because you've tuned to channel 7. Channel 5 has become a dream, has dissolved back into the cosmos. All forms are relative forms, real only within the dream.

Enlightenment doesn't mean that you reject life. Enlightenment means you are standing nowhere. It means you are free of all clinging in life. Now, just to clear up any doubts, I'll tell you from the outset that I am not enlightened. I would be the first to say I was if I were! What I have seen gives me a sense of what is possible, and I'll certainly not settle for anything less. But I am enjoying the course of the journey, patiently watching myself move in that direction. I see a falling away of old stuff all the time and I'm absolutely delighted; the journey is going slow enough for me to enjoy it.

Enlightenment comes in all packages. Many of us have tasted

bliss, but we aren't always living in bliss. Often we are just remembering the moments we were in bliss. To stand up when we are not in bliss and say "I am in bliss" creates a big problem. I have to deal with my own hypocrisy all the time. What I do is make it public. I tell people exactly where I am; this means we can work together as friends on a journey. To stand up and say "I am not in bliss today" without losing face means we have to have a lot of respect for our audience. We've got to see our audience as us, not as them. "Them" are people I'm afraid of, whereas "us" is just family. When everybody is "us," it makes it a lot easier to be ourselves.

There are a lot of things we get trapped in, not just things like anger but "nice" things like doing good, being a helper, or serving needy people. But service in which we are busy identifying with being the servant is just more ego. True compassionate action comes out of the awareness that we are all inseparable. It's not the level where everything dissolves into nothing; it's the level of soul, where we are unique but where we are all part of the same thing, and therefore your suffering is my suffering. There is just suffering, and the suffering awakens the response which people call compassion but which is shared suffering. We are not doing it for ego enhancement, and it's no big deal. It's just an expression of our being.

To bring about a more compassionate and saner society will take a deep shift in consciousness. What will precipitate that shift is in the hands of God. But the deeper my wisdom goes, the more I feel that there are no errors. I'm learning to see the perfection at the same moment that I, as a human being, feel the absolute absurdity and horror and pathology of it all. I'm learning to live with both these planes of consciousness simultaneously: being in the game, and yet seeing it is a game. And the game is scary. Little children get mangled in it, people get cancer, there is suffering and unhappiness. The moment we don't have the balance of seeing it all as an unfolding of law—karmic law or Dharma—we're in trouble.

The path of bhakti is seeing the Beloved in everybody. As we start to experience ourselves as souls, our very way of being becomes an environment in which other people begin to see their own souls. We become an environment in which souls can play together. And more and more we see those souls as just different faces of the Beloved. It's all God at play. We need to train our soul vision so that we look at the world from a soul's point of view. And we need to find soul playmates who look at the world the same way.

The web is so intertwined, so interconnected, that if we live true to our deepest understanding, if we extricate ourselves not from our desires but from our identification with them, then our awareness is spacious enough to hear what is. It will be nice when we can shift from being seekers, from searching for ourselves, to being finders. Why not assume that we have already won the lottery and that we are indeed as beautiful as we hoped we might be (but doubted that we were)? Then we can enjoy the dance of life. The optimum act in this moment arises from hearing what is.

Christina Feldman

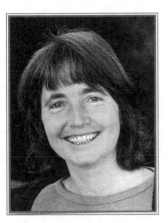

For more than twenty years Christina Feldman has been leading insight meditation retreats, after her own training in Thailand. A deeply compassionate and pragmatic practitioner and teacher, she talks here about the need for acceptance of ourselves and our circumstances. "There are many things we cannot take responsibility for in this world, but the one thing we can be responsible for is a quality of presence in this moment."

Acceptance

Some years ago I was fortunate in being able to visit an island that was promoted as being a kind of paradise. A bit to my surprise I discovered the brochures had not lied. It was beautiful, tropical, lush, and there did not even seem to be anything unpleasant—there were no snakes, wild animals, or hidden dangers. It seemed to be this benevolent and wonderful place, except for one thing. On this island there was a very poisonous kind of tree. There were not that many of these trees, but they were very present on beaches, in parks, and beside sidewalks. We were strongly warned that just one drop of sap from such a tree would burn like acid and be powerful enough to send us into shock.

All this struck me as a little strange. Why not just cut them down? It was not as if the islanders got anything from these trees: they were not used for wood, they bore no edible fruit, and you could not even shelter under them when it was raining. In fact, that was the most dangerous time to be under one, as you could get sapped on. But the islanders did not cut them down. The most they did was to occasionally put a fence around one, and they would almost always hang a sign on them saying Poisonous Tree. But apart from that, the trees were just left to be. So at one point during my stay, I asked one of the islanders, "Why don't you just cut them down?" The reaction was one of puzzlement. "Why would we do that?" the man asked. "They were here before we were and they are part of the landscape of our island. It is up to us to take care around them."

It occurred to me that this is a remarkable analogy for our lives, for the way we relate to our world and to ourselves. Many of us have one or more varieties of poisonous trees in our lives. Sometimes these manifest in times of difficulties, struggle, or conflict: we all experience times of illness or of challenge in our working life; we all have relationships with people who are difficult. Sometimes, too, we carry these poisonous trees within ourselves, in terms of our behavior patterns, fears, or habitual reactions. Sometimes the poisonous trees we meet are ones that are rooted in our past—in memories, images, and experiences—and yet surface over and over again in our present and bring sadness or regret.

But what kind of relationship do we personally have to the poisonous trees in our lives or in ourselves? Can we have a simple acknowledgment and acceptance of them? Are we able to treat them with respect, care, or understanding? Do we recognize that they are a part of our personal landscape? Or is our response to our poisonous trees one of trying to get rid of them? Do we say, "How can I get rid of the people or relationships that irritate or threaten me? How do I get rid of the situation or circumstances that keep disturbing me?" We often look for ways to get rid of our difficulties, and this pursuit is often the searching for an ideal world—an undisturbed place that promises calmness, safety, and pleasure.

Acceptance is the most remarkable and precious gift. To be able to both offer and receive it is truly a blessing. You have probably experienced the power of being accepted by others and the ways in which this created an environment of trust, confidence, and openness. It is in those moments of acceptance that we most easily open and deepen in relationship. Acceptance liberates us to be as we are, the moment to be as it is. It liberates other people to learn their own lessons, to find their own way in an atmosphere of respect and appreciation. Acceptance is a precious gift, yet it is also one of the most elusive of qualities.

When I first went to India, I must confess, I really did not like it at all. In spite of all the romantic stories, there were many things I did not like, and one of these was the fact that it disturbed me so much. India is a place that is filled with the capacity to disturb as it is constantly filled with noise. And I happen to be one of those people who do not do well in noise. So after a few weeks of hiding out in a hotel room in a very noisy city, I fled to the mountains looking for quietness, searching for a place where I could begin my meditation practice, which was why I was in India in the first place. I was pretty sure that my ability to meditate depended on getting rid of any disturbance.

So first I found a home in a small village. This was fine for a while, but then I found there was quite a lot in the village that disturbed me: there were lots of people around, so many dogs, and the coming and going of buses. I decided that there was too much disturbance, so I went higher up the mountain and found a hut in which to live. This was also okay for a while, but then again there were people wandering by who would knock at my door to try to sell me things or ask what I was doing there. So I went still higher up the mountain to find another place to live.

But still I found myself being disturbed! This time I did things like put blankets on the windows to shut out the sun, I used earplugs to shut out the noise, and I did not go outside. Yet still the world managed to intrude. In that part of the Indian mountains there are enormous silver monkeys, and they would come and dance on my roof, which was made of tin. I would sit down to meditate, and there would be this stamping, galloping, and thumping. I could never find earplugs that would shut all this out.

One day I found myself standing outside my hut shouting at the monkeys to go away, to stop disturbing me. Then slowly—and it took a little while—it dawned on me that the monkeys were just being monkeys, that the sun was just being the sun, that sounds were just being sounds, that none of this had any agenda whatsoever to disturb me, that the monkeys did not get up in the morning and think, "Oh, what a good day to go out and get the person trying to meditate." In that moment of stopping and pausing I realized what really disturbed me was my capacity to be disturbed. My capacity, my inclination, my imbalance was finding disturbance in all things.

Three of the primary forces of nonacceptance are aversion, desire or craving, and expectation.

We can have a pretty powerful habit of aversion in our lives. There are the small aversions that can accompany us—the little irritations, complaints, dislikes, and discontents. These are not major dramas; there is nothing life-threatening if the food is too spicy or too bland or if a person in front of us walks too slowly. And yet the mind has these little irritations with which we don't feel at ease in the moment. This is the mosquito level of aversion: the mosquito buzzes around and takes a little bite now and again; we will not die from it, just be slightly uncomfortable.

Then there is another layer of aversion made up of much larger aversions. These are quite harsh. They manifest when we find ourselves inwardly shouting at another person in judgment or feeling resentful and bitter. They are like a small fire within us, not easy to let go of. And we are aware that these layers of aversion separate us from other people and from ourselves. They are the bees or wasps of aversion: they carry something of a sting.

And then there is the monster layer of rage, anger, and hatred. These aversions primarily and most deeply affect our self-image. We know that beneath many of these aversions is the fear of being hurt, abused, or overwhelmed. To understand aversion, we need to go to this level, to the place in ourselves where we carry and manifest fear. Normally we just pay attention to the children of aversion in terms of discontents or judgments; we try to fix things, to avoid our feelings, to appear perfect. We do not often connect or make contact with the roots of that aversion. But aversion can act as a kind of wake-up call to pay attention to our hearts, our feelings, our mind. What is the actual presence of fear in this moment? Where is fear moving me? What am I trying to protect? Where do I fear being hurt? What is that place in me that feels so available yet so vulnerable and that is so easily wounded? In the midst of that which we find most difficult, we will find our balance, strength, and steadiness.

Another of the forces of nonacceptance is the area of craving, wanting or desire, in relationship to sensations and feelings. So often we find ourselves facing the hungriness of the never-enough mind. The nature of craving is separation: the frustration of separation, of always feeling separated from that which we need, depend on, or want in order to be happy. The never-enough mind makes frequent appearances and creates a deep restlessness. And yet the more we want, the more we feel empty, incomplete, or lacking within ourselves. And that feeling of incompleteness sends us fleeing to the next promise, the next thing that we can find or gain.

Can we stay very close to that sense of restlessness? In the midst of restlessness, in the midst of wanting, there is a place where it is important to be still, to be present. It is only when we are still that we begin to listen, to go beneath the restlessness, to question that sense of hunger or lack.

The third area of nonacceptance is in the area of expectation. This has a very strong link to both aversion and wanting. There are very valid expectations we have, ones that are realistic, that have to do with the realities in our lives. And there is also a whole other layer of expectations that have to do with a dissatisfied mind and a hungry heart, that are less valid or realistic.

During my own journey I went to Thailand in order to practice meditation. I had very high expectations that the monastery would be an oasis of peace, respect, and wisdom. The reality was very different. When I finally ended up in a monastery where I decided to stay for awhile, I found myself noticing all the things that were wrong. There were monks who played the radio, monks who were standing around chattering all the time, ones who ate too much at lunchtime, and others who were quite unmindful. What I did not see, of course, were all the monks who were practicing sincerely, who were generous and kind, or who were incredibly silent. Because my expectations were being disappointed, I had this kind of tunnel vision. I did not have any time to meditate because I was too busy criticizing. I quite forgot why I was there, that I had gone to this place in order to practice, in order to cultivate peace. My intention was actually to be awake, but I forgot all about this.

There is a story about a man in Aachan Cha's monastery who did exactly the same things I was doing. He kept complaining to Aachan Cha about why the monks were not better meditators, why they were not more mindful, or why they did not eat less. Aachan Cha said to this man, "You are like somebody that keeps chickens and then goes out in the morning and picks up the droppings instead of the eggs."

In the Tibetan tradition there is a verse that aspiring yogis repeat before they begin to meditate. They say, "Grant that I may be given appropriate difficulties and suffering on this journey so that my heart may be truly awakened and my practice of liberation and universal compassion may be truly fulfilled." This verse is not asking us to be martyrs or to go through unending pain. But it is asking us to bring our aspirations, intention, and intuition into every moment of our lives. Anyone can be accepting when she or he is undisturbed; it is not that difficult to be compassionate when nobody is interfering with what we want, to be loving when we are being flattered, to be forgiving when we have not been really hurt. But in those moments when we are in contact with fear, anger, or uncomfortable feelings, then we are asked to find very deep levels of compassion, acceptance, forgiveness, and understanding. It is in those moments of contact that we can begin to move away from resistance, aversion, or judgment.

This is acceptance: the capacity to stay still in the midst of the difficult and the challenging. There are many things we cannot take responsibility for in this world, but the one thing we can be responsible for is a quality of presence in this moment. We cannot fix or even change other people; we cannot make the world fit into our mold, but we can connect with the quality of presence in this moment. We may need first to take the step of being willing to disengage from the activities of expectation and craving, to step back from acting out our aversions. Once we have stepped back, we can be still and we can listen. Acceptance is not some sort of grandiose romantic notion. It is increasing our capacity to see what is true and to live in harmony with this. There is a wonderful Chinese proverb that says, "When my heart is at peace the world is at peace." This comes through acceptance.

Matthew Fox

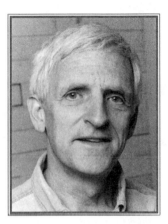

Ordained as a priest in 1967, Matthew Fox took his own path away from the organized church and founded Creation Spirituality, which has touched the hearts of many people worldwide. Here he talks about the philosophy behind Creation Spirituality, which, he states, "is the tradition that Divinity is everywhere, the unity in all things. It recognizes that the Kingdom of God is here among us; we just have to change our perception."

Techno Cosmic Masses

I grew up in Wisconsin, which is a farming state with a lot of trees
and fields and seasons; I loved the experience of wonder and awe at
the sacredness of nature. But I also grew up in a university town
where the political and intellectual dimensions were very palpable. I
entered the Dominican order because they had a tradition that included the intellectual and the aesthetic; Aquinas said that revelation
comes in two volumes, nature and the Bible. But I think that most
seminarians, within a year, have forgotten the nature part and look
exclusively at the book. We have to reconnect with the revelation of
unity in nature. My whole work has been to demonstrate that the
West has a profound mystical tradition: Hildegard of Bingen, Meister
Eckhart, Julian of Norwich, and Aquinas all embodied the mystical
tradition in Christianity. I also work a lot with native peoples, from
the Native Americans to the Aborigines. They make up for what we
are missing in Western theology. They have the deeper traditions that
honor the presence of God in nature and cosmology; they have
prayers and spiritual practices that elicit nature, such as drumming
and dancing.

Most of the mainline churches are so indebted to the academic
definition of theology that they have lost the mystical dimension. It's
one thing to honor the right brain, but you need to keep the left

brain going too. I ask seminarians how many scientists they have on their faculty teaching the wonder and mysticism that is in science, and the creation story of cosmology, or how many artists they have teaching art as meditation. There is a danger that we just talk about mysticism and thereby avoid the experiential dimension.

Prayer or meditation is the practical dimension of spirituality, along with social justice and service. We need both of those. We need prayer and meditation to center our psyche, to cleanse and empty it, to discipline and gear it up; it's like building the muscles of the soul, which get flabby from disuse, especially in our culture, with television and so much distraction coming at us all the time. As we get older, the clarity in our own thinking and creativity is often diminished by this constant input. Meditation is about emptying the mind of images so that we can be present to our own creativity.

Creation Spirituality is the tradition that Divinity is everywhere, the unity in all things. It recognizes that the Kingdom of God is here among us; we just have to change our perception. We are creating a ritual center, where we have what we call Techno Cosmic Masses, drawing on the urban language of the youth with their trance dancing, multimedia, electronic music, and rap poetry and using this to awaken and draw the community together. The service consists of music and dance and the projection of images on the walls and ceilings so that we create a sacred temple. One of our services was on angels, and we had more than five hundred slides of angels and spirits—Native American, Taoist, Buddhist, Hindu, Christian, and Jewish—projected onto the ceilings and walls and we danced in their presence. So even though the services are somewhat recognizable as masses, they include other peoples' spiritual traditions. We celebrated another around the sacredness of the body; we projected twenty-eight organs of the body on the walls and we all danced among them. The masses are about recovering a sense of the sacred in every aspect of our lives.

One nineteen-year-old Jewish man said after one of our masses that he had had the most powerful religious experience of his life, and a fifty-year-old woman said that it was the most expansive experience her Protestant soul had ever undergone. A forty-two-year-old woman had tears coming down her cheeks during the dancing; she said, "This is a language in which I can pray with my teenage son." Up until that time she had felt that her son didn't have a language for faith or prayer.

A community needs to meditate and to worship together. It needs to have ritual because most of the rituals today are very boring, they are not working, they are not reaching people's hearts. If we can find ways, especially through the new technology, of making worship interesting again, then this is a gift to the community. Every community needs to celebrate; it needs to do healing, to reach its down-and-outs, its young people, its unemployed, and even its overemployed. There is pain at all levels of society, and we have to help get it out. How many rituals do we have in which people can moan and wail their grief together about the loss of our environment? We always have a part of our masses that is wailing, and afterward people often say that is the most powerful part because they have never before been invited to grieve in a group. They did all their grieving alone, and that is not healing enough.

The work of compassion is the culmination of the spiritual journey as understood in the Creation Spirituality tradition; there is no conclusion to the journey without it. Many people in the New Age movement pay so much attention to the light that often they ignore the shadow, the darkness, and the injustice. A healthy spirituality has to deal with both. Mysticism is about life, whereas the prophetic tradition is about saying no to the injustice, trying to enter the darkness and do something about it. This combination of mysticism and prophecy is the nature of healthy spirituality.

The journey of the universe puts our own journey in context. The universe has been on a journey for fifteen billion years; it began smaller than a pinprick, and now it's very vast. So individually we are each a part of a much bigger journey but only a very recent part—just one million years old, maybe. So much was done on our behalf, in terms of Earth's being possible. It took one billion years to get the ozone layer just right, and now we're punching big holes into it because we are oblivious of the blessing and the grace that creation has given to us. The other creatures, from what we know of them, seem much more at home in the universe; we seem to be the ones who want to blow things up and do damage. We are part of a very big journey, and we should behave as honored guests on the path.

The purpose of the journey is to contribute to the whole. And that is a role to celebrate. Our responsibility is to celebrate and praise the creative universe for what has been accomplished, while paying attention to the suffering and pain that are also present. Obviously the ecological crisis, beyond any ideology, is the number-one moral issue of our times. How do we heal the holes in the ozone layer? How do we heal the rain forests which are being torn down at the rate of one acre a second? How do we heal the fisheries in the ocean that are being fished out? We have to change our ways, to reinvent the way we exist on the planet. We are destroying 27,000 species a year. At this rate of destruction, in fifty years there will be no species.

Even if we do tear down trees for wood or kill animals to eat, it should be done with reverence and not out of greed or for an exclusive economic goal, because the profit motive is not adequate to the human soul; it's not why we're here. We are here for a broader purpose than just profit. Profit is only about diminishing what we bequeath to future generations while giving a few people a lot of money. Too few win. What can you buy that's more beautiful than the grace of a healthy forest?

I feel moral outrage at the state of the world, but that's all part of grief. The first level of grief is anger. And you have to go deeper into the rage and go into the sorrow, which is the second stage of grief, and deal with that too. And then you have to go into the emptying, the letting go, the third stage of grief. There is a relationship between beauty and terror. The more you connect to the beauty and grace of existence, the more aware you are of the terror of death and destruction. If you develop an inner life, then your soul finds space for the experience of awe, wonder, beauty, and grace, as well as the experience of darkness and letting go.

Anger is a very important passion that is directly related to our capacity to love. We get angry because something we cherish is threatened. Anyone who is not angry is either not in love or not in touch with what they say they love. Thomas Aquinas said that a trustworthy person is angry at the right people and for the right reasons and expresses it in the appropriate manner and for the appropriate length of time. The most important point is the appropriate length of time, for the danger with anger is getting attached to it. When you start living your life on anger, then you fall into bitterness, and your creativity stops. Aquinas said that nothing creative gets done without anger. I think that anger is sinful when it becomes an attachment, a whole worldview, but in itself anger is a very healthy emotion to pay attention to. It tells us about the work we have to do, and it gives us energy to get it done.

There is a lot of anger in young people. One way it expresses itself is in self-destruction, such as indirect suicide through unsafe sex, drugs or alcohol, or driving while drinking. Anger becomes self-destructive when it is turned inward. One of the best ways to heal anger is to let it out, to turn it into theater, rap, music, dance, art, to put it into the body, to tell the story that makes you angry in a form that you can tell it. Another thing to do with anger is ritual. This puts anger in the context of the universe. Without a cosmology, you can't deal with your pain or your anger. You keep it inside or you take pills or drink or you numb it through television or shopping. All these addictions that Western societies are so good at selling constitute pseudoways of dealing with pain or anger. When your heart breaks, you have to take that break to the universe. Without a cosmology it just gets bottled up inside; this I think is the cause of a lot of violence.

Ritual is the traditional way of giving people the sense of the universe and cosmology. Native people teach their young to live in the universe through dance, story, and drumming. In fact, drumming is an ancient way to pray. The heartbeat that you heard from your mother for nine months in the womb is also the heartbeat of the Creator, of the universe itself. When you beat a drum, you're beating an animal's hide, so you're riding on that animal into the land of grief and anger. If you do that on a daily basis, going into grief work and anger work, it becomes very healing.

There are three reasons for the "drug quest" in the West. One is to experience transcendence and the second is to numb the pain, which includes anger. Community experience is the third motive. But there are more creative ways of dealing with pain besides doing drugs. Through our Techno Cosmic Masses we are trying to show the young people in the rave movement that it doesn't have to be about drugs, that you can get high and have transcendent experiences through cosmology and spirituality.

I think we have to take a hard look at our inner lives and bring them to bear on our outer work. We have to bring our joy, our wonder, and our awe alive first, and we have to bring them to our work. We have to do it in our relationships, in our marriages, in our parenting, in the election of our government officials, in our ecological awareness, and in doing business. Where is the joy in our work? If we can't answer that question, then we have a job but we don't have work, because work should be about joy; it should stem from the heart, and the heart desires joy. We have a right to joy in this world. The world is not just a place for expiating our sins; it should be a place of happiness.

The very structures we have in our workplaces are not working. As E. F. Schumacher said, they are killing the soul. If our body gets injured at work, we have insurance, but if our soul gets injured, we're on our own. We go home and watch television because we're so numb, or we go to a therapist because the soul is so damaged. The two industries that have grown up as a response to the industrial revolution are therapy and entertainment; both are about the soul being wounded. I know a priest on the East Coast at a prestigious medical school who was hired just to live in the dormitory to prevent suicides. The year before, four students had committed suicide and ten had tried and failed. Idealistic young people who want to be healers start training, and within a year they want to commit suicide. What's going on here? And instead of questioning that maybe this education thing is being done wrong, they hire priests to prowl the corridors.

When people don't have a cosmology, they get pathological. There is little wisdom in our medical schools, in academia, in our education; we're just in pursuit of knowledge. And knowledge alone is very dangerous; it has been the passion of Western civilizations, but it has now run its course and become destructive. And what we have as a result is stress. I think a university has become like a strainer that strains the soul out. We're not going to reinvent our work or professions until we reinvent education, because that's where the damage begins.

To reinvent education, we have started a University of Spirituality in downtown Oakland. It is very exciting—trying to create urban spirituality and to reawaken the connection between spirituality, work, and daily life. Most universities have lost a sense of the universe; they don't have this perception of wisdom or celebration, the joy of learning that ought to be a part of the educational experience. On our faculty we have cosmologists, scientists, and artists; we have indigenous people teaching everything from Yoga to African dance and drumming; and we bring these traditions together in a way that is really powerful.

Do you see your life as a blessing and a gift? This is the main thing now for me. I was blessed because when I was twelve, I had polio. I had people telling me I would never walk again, but I did; I got my legs back. I thought I would never take my legs for granted again, and that was so important. If you've ever seen a dying person, you'll know that the breath is where it all ends. So we shouldn't take the breath for granted; we shouldn't take anything for granted. We have to reassess our basic attitudes, to see that our lives are true gifts.

Rupert Sheldrake

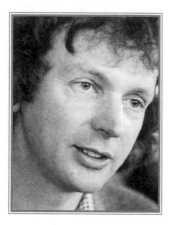

A scientist and revolutionary thinker, Rupert Sheldrake has often challenged the scientific world. In his contribution he explores the relationship of science and spirit, which at one time were not seen as separate but as two facets of the same whole. "The theologians have contracted from the universal to a limited human sphere, while the scientists have purged the universe of anything to do with higher meaning."

Our Cosmic Dimension

Back in the Middle Ages there was a recognition that the realms of philosophy, nature, science, and theology were distinct yet compatible. The Middle Ages inherited its philosophy from the ancient Greeks, particularly Aristotle and Plato. The genius of St. Thomas Aquinas and his contemporaries was the ability to combine classical philosophy and cosmology with Christian theology. This understanding made it clear that although science, philosophy, and religion occupied separate realms, as they came from separate sources, they were also in keeping with each other: Christian theology fitted with a greater cosmology, as seen in angels or a respect for Nature. The official philosophy was one of Christian animism, with Nature as a living organism, Earth as alive, animals and plants as having souls. The English word animal comes from the Latin *anima,* which means "soul." Such animism was the official doctrine taught in the medieval universities.

The idea of the soul as being "that which animates living beings" included the belief that even the planets have intelligence. The pagan understanding was that the planets were gods—such as Venus, Mercury, or Mars—but the Christian view was that they were not so much gods as angels—beings with their own minds and intelligences. In this way the many gods of the ancient world became the angels of the Christian world. So the people of that time lived in a world full of living beings: some at higher levels than the human realm, such as angels, others at lower levels, such as animals and plants. This can be seen in such Gothic cathedrals as Exeter or Chartres, in which there is a fantastic integration of nature and cosmos: There are green men surrounded by foliage and natural forms, and there are gargoyles, guardian spirits, and demons—all integrated into the structure of this divine temple of worship, so a link is created between earth and heaven. The medieval cathedrals, therefore, show us how this synthesis was a living reality.

However, with the sixteenth century came the Protestant Reformation. At that time there were hundreds of seasonal festivals, local saints, and pilgrimages to all sorts of ancient power spots such as sacred mountains or wells. There was the cult of the Holy Mother, which the Protestants rightly identified as a thinly disguised goddess cult, and the cult of the Blessed Virgin. Whereas the Catholic Church had embraced and incorporated all these aspects of paganism, the Protestants were purists—narrow, rather scholarly figures—and they realized that historically these things were not Christian. They wanted to purify the religion, and so they threw out all the pagan aspects. What was left was a religion centered on human beings and their relationship to God. Nature was not included; it was seen as just a kind of backdrop to the drama of fall and redemption, played out between man and God.

This human-centeredness was called humanism. It was involved with the whole tradition of human abilities, literature, and culture, which in its secular form became the dominant spirit of the modern age. Humanism is a form of speciesism; it puts humans very much above the rest of creation, treating human beings as the only conscious beings in the universe. Angels are seen as just a kind of medieval fantasy or at best a poetic fiction, and the idea of innumerable forms of consciousness above the human level is dispensed with. The whole of the universe is inanimate, soulless; all that is left is the rational conscious mind located somewhere in the head.

In the early seventeenth century a peaceful coexistence was arrived at, a deal done between science and religion to try to minimize conflict: science got the whole of the universe—all the stars, the planets, and the earth and all the animals and plants, as well as the human body—while religion got the human soul, morality, ethics, redemption, and eternal life. So the sphere of religion was immensely contracted. We see this reflected in more recent Protestant churches in which the focus is on the Bible, on man, and on sin and redemption. There is a greater emphasis on Jesus—the human side of God—in contrast to the medieval view in which God was seen as the God of the entire universe, the Holy Spirit pervading nature.

The idea of seeing living organisms as machines was developed by Descartes through a vision he had in 1619. He believed that the whole world was an inanimate machine, the whole of nature soulless, animals and plants mere mechanical structures. The only thing left with souls were human beings. But even they no longer had a "body soul." Previously, it was thought that human souls had a "vegetative soul" which organized the body, just as plants had a soul which gave shape to their bodies and was concerned with healing and regeneration; then there were the "animal soul" which gave human beings their animal and instinctive nature and the "rational" or "intellectual soul" which gave human beings their conscious mind and higher mental faculties. The traditional view was not that the soul was in the body but that the body was in the soul; the soul both encompassed and shaped the body. But after Descartes, the body was seen as just a machine with a rational intellect in the head, somehow interacting with the machinery of the brain.

In this way soul became something that only human beings had, and it became equated with the rational mind. I believe that this contraction of the soul is coming to an end as science grows beyond the idea that the universe is just a machine. Now we are seeing the whole cosmos as evolutionary—having started very small with the big bang—growing from less than the size of the head of a pin. It is more like a developing organism than a machine. At the same time, the old idea of rigid determinism has now given way to indeterminism, to spontaneity and chaos. As we break out of the old mechanistic view, science gives us a vastly expanded view of the cosmos, with galaxies and black holes—creativity on a cosmic scale that goes beyond mere matter.

Meanwhile, institutional religion is not doing too well as many people are feeling the need to reconnect with nature. This can be seen in the ecological movement which is a direct recognition that humankind is a part of Gaia, the living earth. It suggests that we have to go beyond the narrow focus of purely human concerns. Certainly, the human realm is important, but to make it our sole focus is the reason why, I believe, so many things have gone wrong. The modern world is based on an extreme exaggeration of the human at the expense of the recognition that we are interdependent with nature, the earth, and the whole cosmos.

I believe we need to recover a sense of our cosmic dimension. We need to ask, if God in heaven is the traditional view, does that mean God is in the whole universe? What does a Divine presence in the universe mean? If the angels are celestial presences, then what role do the angels play in the galaxies and the stars? If they are the intelligences of galaxies and the minds of stars, then what are all those minds doing out there? This is a whole realm that neither theologians, who have been locked into a medieval worldview in relation to angels, nor scientists have considered. The theologians have contracted from the universal to a limited human sphere, while the scientists have purged the universe of anything to do with higher meaning. I am convinced that the way forward is to break out of these narrow limitations, to try to build bridges between these two areas.

Angels have become fairly incredible to people since the mechanistic worldview came in: there's not much room for angels; we have a rather collapsed view of religion in which there are human beings and God with nothing in between, and the whole of nature is just a kind of backdrop. But it was never conceived that way in any of the traditional religions; there has always been a big role for angels and other forms of intelligence between the human and the Divine realms. The traditional view is that angels are derived from God and share in Divine aspects of consciousness but that they are more limited forms of intelligence than the Divine; they have their own particular differentiation.

I've never personally met an angel, and I don't expect that angels really go around with wings or halos. Even medieval writers believed this was a symbolic description of how they have the power of moving at the speed of thought. I see angels on a cosmic level, as the intelligences that pervade the entire universe and guide the evolutionary process. There are many levels of angels to do with galaxies, solar systems, and planets—the creative intelligences that pervade all nature. Then there are angels that are particularly concerned with guiding our life on Earth, and I think the way they work is mainly as creative spirits. A lot of the modern interest in angels concerns a very practical, personalized approach, such as when your car breaks down on the freeway and then suddenly this mysterious figure arrives, mends it, and disappears. That kind of angel I've never encountered. But I do experience a sense of guidance in my own life and think of that as being angelic. I think that there are many forms of differentiated consciousness, and the ones that are above the human level are, by definition, angelic. Some of them may be associated with stars or planets, and some may not.

The traditional view in Christianity is that the Divine nature is threefold, that Divine consciousness is not undifferentiated but contains an internal differentiation of consciousness seen in the Holy Trinity. There is what is known and there is the means of knowing. There may be forms of consciousness that are contentless, but most of our experience of consciousness is consciousness with content. In the Trinity, the Father is the ground of consciousness, while the Son is that which is known, which also knows the Father. The interim notion between the two, that which connects them, is the Holy Spirit.

I believe that Divine consciousness is more like an organism, more like a community, than an isolated individual. Love is built into the very nature of Divine consciousness, for if the Divine is seen as an isolated individual consciousness, then it would be self-love which is narcissistic, whereas community implies selfless love. In the same way, I believe that the spiritual life is not just an individual matter; it's also a collective matter, and it's very important to have a collective expression. This is why I go to church. There are many individualistic ways of practicing spiritual life, but such individual models are, to me, just a reflection of an individualistic, consumer society, in which everyone is fragmented and there is no social cohesion. Traditional societies always have collective rituals, collective expressions of their spiritual life. We see this in nature, such as bees working in a hive for the common good. Altruism has a strong biological basis; it's not just a human thing.

In the human realm, the higher forms of altruism depend on a broader vision, a sense that one is part of a larger whole that connects to the earth and the cosmos. It is this larger vision that provides the basis for selfless behavior. We already have a much greater awareness of our interconnectedness simply through modern communications—telephones, the Internet, and travel—and we are far more aware of the many different cultural and religious traditions. On the one hand we can say that this communication brings us into the presence of the riches of all the world, but on the other it means we can have an increase in the dominance of some cultures over others. At the moment, the dominant culture seems to be that of Hollywood, as hundreds of TV channels rain down on India, China, and the third world. There is a cultural imperialism happening which is not a celebration of richness and diversity but rather the imposition of the lowest common denominator.

Our scientific picture of the universe shows how we are related to everything else in the entire cosmos. Every part of my body and every part of yours has the history of the whole cosmos within it, which links up to the entire development of all nature. In the Middle Ages they had a very limited cosmology, with Earth at the center of a series of spheres and the stars on the outermost sphere— a cozy, small cosmos. We now have this unimaginably vast cosmos with fifteen billion years of cosmic evolution behind it—a vastly greater scope for spiritual and religious imagination. At the same time that science has given us this previously unimaginable sense of the vastness of the universe, it has also given us the whole microscopic realm—levels within levels. I think part of our task is to recognize this vastness which science has opened up and to try to come to terms with what it means to be alive in the midst of it.

One thing science shows us is that there is an incredible variety of creativity and diversity in the natural world—a fantastic creativity in everything—which I see as Divine in source. It gives me a sense that excessive preoccupation with the merely human level is very provincial, that this awareness of the vastness of things can give us the perspective that our role is not as big as we would like it to be. One of the great challenges for the future is finding ways of linking to other forms of consciousness. I don't have much time for UFOs and alien abductions, but I do think that there are many forms of consciousness in the universe beyond the human level. If we are going to contact them, then we will do it not through spaceships and hardware but through something more like telepathy.

The next frontier is about making contact not just with other forms of consciousness but also with the Divine consciousness. After all, if people see the purpose of life as being the evolution of human consciousness, then it is hard to believe that the purpose of the entire universe is just to have human consciousness on this planet and this one alone. And if it is, then what is the rest of the universe for, with its innumerable galaxies and so forth? Is it just there to enter into the catalogues of astronomers? I cannot believe that it is just to be a backdrop. So if there is a purpose in the evolution of consciousness, it cannot just be of human consciousness on this planet; it must also be something to do with the consciousness of the rest of the universe.

The way we are linked together in a collective human consciousness gives us a responsibility that goes beyond the merely personal. What we do and say can affect people throughout the world. Even what we think can affect other people. So we are both collectively and individually responsible to Earth. I do not doubt for a minute that Gaia will survive. The survival of the human race is much more questionable. But if human civilization as we know it does collapse, then it is probably a good thing for most of the species on the planet. There is a difference between the survival of human civilization and the survival of the natural world. Even if human beings do their very worst, life will go on. If you go to Chernobyl, right in the most contaminated areas, there are plants growing and birds singing. They may be more muted than usual, but life is going on.

International forums, even the most high-minded like the Rio Summit, have an extremely limited capacity to change things; committees of politicians, academics, or businesspeople do not seem to be a way of saving the world. They do have a role to play and it is important not to neglect this role, but it is not going to be our salvation. Salvation is going to depend on forms of consciousness higher than our own, so I think we are going to have to rely on prayer and guidance to find our way forward. We have to look beyond the human realm to find inspiration for the future: to God, the angels, the saints, and the creative spirit that work in such mysterious ways.

Kittisaro and Thanissara

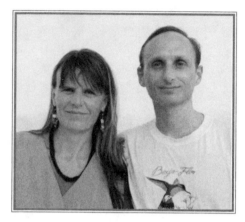

*A*merican-born Kittisaro was a Buddhist monk for fifteen years, and Thanissara, from England, was a nun for twelve years. Now married, they share with us a model of how to apply profound spiritual truths in a world of conflict and confusion. "We have the choice to create our world out of fear, aversion, and greed," they say, "or to see the potential to create it out of wisdom, joy, and sensitivity."

Faith in an Uncertain World

The blue sky stretches out, farther and farther,
The daily sense of failure goes away,
The damage I have done to myself fades,
A million suns come forth with light,
When I sit firmly in that world.

KABIR

There are many things to worry about in this troubled world. We write this while staying at a friend's house in Johannesburg, and we could easily be anxious or fearful in recollecting that this house has been burgled fourteen times in five months and in being amid the senseless killings and constant threats of violence, fear, and despair. What is the answer? Higher walls, more razor wire, better electronic gates, smarter alarms, more powerful guns? Although these "solutions" may allow us to think we are safer or more secure, the fear of "them out there" and what they might do still lurks in the shadows of our minds.

This feeling of uncertainty and anxiety around the world is highly accentuated here in South Africa, in a post-apartheid society whose emergence from the old repressive regime is threatened by an alarming increase in crime and violence. The future is always uncertain, especially at such times of great transition. This fear of the unknown can either lead us to grasp more tightly at old ways of being or be an opportunity to open our minds to other dimensions of possibility. Perhaps a starting point is the inquiry into where we find stability and some kind of reference point for our lives. Rather than trying to freeze life into a manageable concept, there is the potential to learn to be at ease with the uncertainty by deepening a sense of refuge in the innate awareness of mind itself.

We abandon this innate awareness when we get lost in the beguiling appearance of our thoughts, fears, and desires. The manifestation of our world is then re-created moment by moment out of fantasy and confusion. To save this world from those conditions which most of us abhor—violence, anguish, cruelty, tyranny—we need to understand them. How can we know the world unless we connect with it through mindful attention and clear comprehension? With the discipline of attention applied in a sustained way to the moments of our experience, we begin to see the needless tensions and suffering we create. In this way of self-responsibility we have the choice to create our world out of fear, aversion, and greed or to see the potential to create it out of wisdom, joy, and sensitivity.

We all know we are supposed to be kind, generous, and loving, but without wisdom we have no way of dealing with negativity and pain. Our modern culture tends not to be a wise culture. It is intelligent, powerful, and ambitious, but it often lacks depth of understanding, partly because we deny so many of the realities of life and death. Inevitably, it is the experience of pain that brings the attention needed for deeper inquiry; without understanding suffering, we never realize the end of suffering. We may try all manner of ways to feel fulfilled and happy, and yet when our pain is denied, our suffering becomes more acute. Rather than reacting blindly to pain, if we can open to the experience of suffering with mindful attention, we hold the key to transformation; as we contemplate our suffering, the door of wisdom begins to open. Even at our darkest hour there is a real potential for change.

We can begin this way of intelligent kindness very simply by being in touch with the feeling of the body, without judgment, allowing the heart-mind to be steadied by the rhythm of the breath. As we learn to steady the mind, we unexpectedly discover a home within awareness that is restful and healing. The heart brightens and finds its inner radiance and tranquillity as it contemplates the simplicity of the body. When the mind is confused, we tend to generate more confusion in trying to overcome our limitations. However, when we remember the refuge of the heart, we can turn to the moment in a subtle gesture of acceptance and trust. The body, the breath, a sound, even the troubling mood itself can take us home if we receive it patiently and respectfully. When each one of us— uniquely positioned in the changing world of form—befriends the heart, we can transform blind reactivity into compassionate response.

Though most of us do not know how the future will unfold, we can at least understand that our present choices influence whatever comes into being. Our capacity for mindful attention, based in awareness, allows for a more creative and wise choice in the way we respond. The Buddha's famous statement that "mind is the forerunner of all things" demonstrates that the results we experience are the direct outcome of the intentions on which we act. Similarly, the beautiful poem by Kabir that introduces this piece gives us hope that however the past has been, there is always the potential for change and redemption. But how do we learn to "sit firmly in that world of a million suns"? Perhaps, as we see the law of karma more clearly, we begin to understand the relationship between the energy of mind and its projections onto the world around us. As the contemplation of this ancient law matures, we also come to know that we have the power either to generate or to alleviate suffering. No longer do we act just for our own interests; rather we naturally take into consideration the interconnectedness of all things.

When the mind desperately seeks stability and protection for "me" in the infinitely complicated realms of "what if," we become more and more disconnected from how it really is, and so fear grows. Over the years both of us have been learning to trust an abiding in truth. This doesn't mean finding solace in convincing ourselves that I am right and you are wrong or tenaciously clinging to my opinion of how it is or how it should be. Abiding in truth is finding our home in awareness. Here we acknowledge the suchness of our experience—the changing circumstances within the flow of life and the timeless sense of presence that is awareness itself.

Through this way of inner listening, we contemplate. What am I protecting? What am I afraid of? Who am I anyway? When the heart asks these questions, old assumptions can be revealed for what they are: false views, mistaken attitudes, illusions not in accord with the truth of this moment. What seems real or unreal to us is directly dependent on the quality of our attention. If we never question our assumptions, then the "truth" of our world is just a perpetual reflection of distorted views and opinions. Consequently, we live in a dream and complain that life is unfair. How can life be satisfactory if we are constantly longing for it to be other than the way it is?

Awareness is not a possession. When everything is bathed in its purifying radiance, the myth of ownership dissolves. When we trust in awareness—that inner listening—as a refuge, then we see directly the changing insubstantial nature of all thoughts. Though the language of self splits the seamlessness of experience into us and them, in the truth of awareness itself all things merge. Mind and body, you and me, life and death, all duality finds a common ground in the pure heart. From this perspective, instead of a sense of "me" going through life, we realize that time and the flow of life are constantly appearing and dissolving within the mind of awareness itself. Here is just the present stillness, the silent vastness, the intimate and transcendent heart.

For so long we have tried to find what we are amidst, the myriad bundle of our daily experiences, and we are frustrated, ever on the move, attempting to maintain the illusion of solidity. We try to avoid the reality of constant change and uncertainty by holding to views about who we are or about how life should be. In letting go of this powerful tendency, we enter the mystery of awareness in which there are no boundaries. With the open-eyed innocence of a child, humbly allowing life to reveal itself, we discover peace. Letting go reveals a lightness of heart in which fear, worry, and hate are received and transformed into trust, patience, and love. Many mystical traditions have described this realization as the Kingdom, Salvation, Nibbana, the Beloved, or Our True Home.

The following poem came to Kittisaro during a year of silence in a small forest hut while a monk in England. Although not well in body at that time, there was an amazement at the beauty of the heart in remembering its true abiding. How easy it is to forget. May all of us, little by little, patiently learn to rejoice in coming home. When we abide in awareness, we put down the heavy burden of ownership. We awaken into that world of a million suns.

Faith
Trust is precious
A treasure trove of gold.
Guard it with all your heart
And you'll never grow old.

It's not a question of this or that
Believed or disbelieved,

But rather letting where you're at
Be silently received.

The heart of faith
The heart that knows
Leaves no trace
And neither comes nor goes.

Stephen and Martine Batchelor

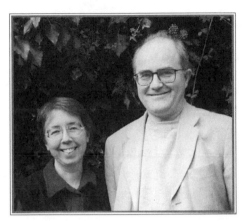

uthors Stephen and Martine Batchelor each lived the monastic Buddhist life for more than ten years, before disrobing and marrying. Now they are directors of the Sharpham College for Buddhist Studies in Devon, England. In the following piece, they discuss issues that revolve around being human and the purpose of life. As Stephen says, "Being fully human means living a life that is, as much as is possible, consciously responding to every facet of one's existence."

Faith, Questioning, and Togetherness

STEPHEN What is it to be a human being? This is the primary question. What does it mean? I don't think it's the sort of question that has an answer hidden away in some mystical realm. Its answer isn't something that will lead us to some final understanding. Of course we would like to have an answer, but we can also block out or forget the primacy of the question. The question relates to the sheer mystery of being, that ultimately we cannot know through intellect or through philosophy, psychology, or religion; there is no final answer. If we use the idea of a spiritual path, then it must be a process of staying with the question, living life out of that question in such a way that keeps the question alive while not allowing it to paralyze or overwhelm us in any way.

So the spiritual path is a way of life that starts by acknowledging and accepting the situation we're in, with our eyes open. It's an honesty with ourselves, an honesty with life; it's facing up to the fact that we have been born and will die. Our way of life then becomes a response to the dilemma of being human. Many people never live their lives in response to the primary questions that life presents, but rather they work out strategies of being successful or strategies of being a particular kind of person. This cuts them off from an authentic response to what life offers in its primary form. To me, being fully human means living a life that is, as much as is possible, consciously responding to every facet of my existence.

MARTINE I would say that the spiritual path is a practice, an action. It's what you do, how you live, how you relate to other people, how you relate to yourself. It is the guiding principle. In a way, what we call spirituality is the inner part, which helps us to relate better to the outer part, so there is no disconnection; rather there is a unity of ourselves and the world. We do need a certain guide or map. We can take any path, but it might not lead anywhere. We can also get stuck in the map, in the details, and then we lose sight of the journey. The aim is to develop fully as a human being and, within that development, to cultivate as much wisdom and compassion as we can until such states become more natural, more evident.

I am aware that the body ends, that I shall die. What is most important for me is my relationship with the world, with people, with an awareness of what is going on in my mind. How do I react? What leads me to do what I do? I want to notice this and to try to transform it so that it is more wise and more compassionate.

STEPHEN The question of life is not just one single thing but a metaphor for everything that is perplexing, puzzling, confusing, and overwhelming. Wisdom and compassion are the twin tracks in which we live out our response to this question. Wisdom, or intelligence, is the capacity to recognize the different facets of this question; compassion is the way in which we respond to the fact that our lives are not solitary and isolated events, that we don't just live entirely in our own isolation but that we are at the same time participants in a shared reality. So intelligence is the way we come to terms with the mystery of our own existence, and compassion is the way we respond to the mystery of being with others.

The two go together as metaphors of that primary polarity of existence, of being alone and being with others. To be alive is to have responses to the questions that life gives us in every moment, in terms of our own mind, our own experience, our own consciousness; it is also in the participatory engagement in that which is "not me," not my mind, not my private experience but which I share with others—people, animals, environment, biosphere, and universe.

MARTINE In all of us there is the capacity to be compassionate, because otherwise how could we create compassion? Compassion is not something that we create from nothing; it is something we reinforce, cultivate, and develop. We do have it to start with. There is this natural, intuitive ability to come out of ourselves, but at the same time there is this very strong impulse to protect ourselves, to be fearful of the world, and so to repress our compassionate impulse. Developing compassion is realizing that it is not so fearful out there, that we do not need to put up all these barriers.

STEPHEN Why is it that people generally admired Mother Teresa? Is it not because she triggered something that we recognize in ourselves as being more real, more true? If we are honest with our response to such people, then there is a spark of that within us, and that spark is what has to be cultivated. However, the reality is that we may get inspired one moment and have a genuine feeling of compassion, but the next day we're feeling a bit depressed or irritated and our compassion has vanished. There is an innate ability to feel these things and to see clearly, but there is also an enormous force of habit and conditioning, both psychological and social, that encourages us to look after ourselves first. The practice of compassion is in consciously seeking ways to nurture that natural tendency, which at times may be a rather forced exercise but ultimately awakens our innate wisdom.

MARTINE   Suppose something terrible happens, whether to ourselves or to someone else. Very quickly we say, "This is terrible; this is awful. The person who did this is very bad." Wisdom then leads us to question what happened, while compassion asks what happened for the person who did it and what happened for the person who received it; there is compassion for both the people involved. We don't condone what the perpetrator did, but she or he is still a human being. To me, the challenge of wisdom is compassion. Instead of saying, "The person who did this is terrible; get rid of her or him," we ask can we do anything about it? Can we help that person not to do it again? Can we help the person who suffered not to suffer so much? In the moment of compassion for another, we break out of our isolation.

Awareness can appear to be like a little person sitting on your shoulder telling you what to do and how to do it. I feel that awareness is closer to intuition. Awareness is knowing something totally in that moment and seeing everything in it, instead of denying the reality. Most of the time there is a story line in our head, and we don't realize that we do what we do because of the story line. We have the capacity to be aware, to be conscious, to look at something, to pay attention, but generally not for very long. Our awareness is very fleeting. What is going on in this moment, this being, this totality, this world? In order to have honesty, we have to accept ourselves, we have to accept our reality; otherwise we are deluded.

STEPHEN   Honesty also has a lot to do with being able to acknowledge that we really don't know. To be honest with ourselves means having to let go of a lot of assumptions, inherited beliefs, and religious beliefs. Being honest means always questioning whatever comes up, and this requires awareness and acceptance, but also it requires the humility to say, "I do not know." I think it is in the depth of that not knowing, of opening to that not knowing, that we are most honest with ourselves. "I don't know" is often seen as a sign of failure. But, if that not knowing is operating in a context of a still, aware, accepting consciousness of the situation we are in at any given moment, then that not knowing is rich and alive with perplexity. The world becomes a question; it doesn't become something that is given and self-evident. If you have a question about something, then you don't know something. You can't say, "I am questioning my existence" and at the same time believe that you know the answer. It's a deep not knowing. This not knowing goes right down into the very depths of the spiritual traditions, but that dimension is often lost because it is far more useful for religions to operate within schemes of belief or pretenses of knowing.

Faith is a sense of confidence that we can respond to life in a much more fulfilling and illuminating way than we habitually do. If we didn't have that faith, then we would not do anything. Faith is believing that things can be other than they are now. I have faith in the fact that I don't always have to cling to the belief that I know something. I can have the faith to live not from that vantage point. So any meaningful human activity is driven by a degree of faith that something else is possible.

MARTINE It's faith in human potential. It's not that you believe in, or have faith in, something outside of yourself, but it's the faith that there is a potential within you that you can develop. It's not that you abstractly believe in something because somebody told you so or it's a good idea or it looks pretty. Faith is very intrinsic.

STEPHEN There is the paradox that faith and doubt are always together, polarities that do not deny each other. Within the context of lived experience, both our questions and the faith that some response to those questions is possible go hand in hand. If you think of belief, it is a very rigid, fixed structure that you cling to, and the opposite is disbelief. We adopt beliefs in order to overcome the difficulty of living with questions, whereas faith and questioning go hand in hand.

Belief is the assumption that there are certain metaphysical claims about truth or reality that we have to take on board in order to engage in a spiritual way of life. Belief is the idea that unless you believe in God, in a multiplicity of lifetimes, or in the enlightenment of the guru, you will have no basis on which to proceed. These are things which we can neither prove nor disprove but which are somehow required by religious institutions as a prerequisite for being part of their communities. That sort of belief is very often at odds with an authentic questioning and response to human existence. Faith is that you have the potential to live with and respond to life in a way that can make a difference but you don't have any fixed idea of what that difference is. Faith does not have any expectations, whereas belief is often the prerequisite for expectations.

Each person has to figure out a response that is true to his or her own situation, while also taking into account the repercussions that every action has across the globe. It cannot be just a self-centered response anymore, for the simple reason that we know how interdependent the world is. We each need to recognize what our skills, strengths, and gifts are, and the challenge of the imagination is how we can use those skills in a way that may make a difference beyond our own immediate circle and perhaps also have repercussions even further afield.

It may be that we sense our isolation to be the primary reality. But if that is the case, then it is useful to recollect that although one does have an experience that is utterly one's own, that experience of one's aloneness is always operative within a simultaneous experience of togetherness. Even if we are living in isolation, we are still speaking to ourselves through a language that is not our own. Moreover, our bodies are not our own; they were given to us through a combination of the cells of our parents. The air we breathe is not our own; it belongs to all of us equally. And the food we eat is not our own; it comes from the earth. So although we have a subjective conviction that "I am just me and I am cut off from the rest of the world," this is simply not true. And at the same time it is equally untrue to say that we are just dissolved in a kind of ecosphere or something and that there is nothing distinctive about each of us. Of course there is. So we have to come to terms with the great paradox of our individual uniqueness and of our utter generality.

Rabbi Zalman Schachter-Shalomi

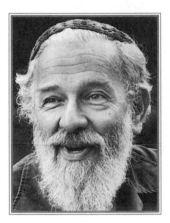

Reb Zalman is a well-loved teacher, writer, and pioneer in Jewish spiritual revival. In his piece he focuses on the spiritual journey and, in particular, the need for spiritual sharing and community. "We have to learn ways of more meaningful collaboration," he says. "On reflection, we must become aware that we need most urgently to get together about getting it together."

A Spirituality of Togetherness

Where do we find spirituality? Like faith, which people loosely speak of having, it is not a thing. We don't find it in only one place, such as a church or synagogue. It's not like I'm collecting butterflies and I have it there—it's a that, it measures so, and it looks like this—because that doesn't show the living experience. My spiritual home is not an object; it is a living experience. And, just as a living being, it is subject to changes.

Every religion is experiencing a shift in consciousness and is having to find new ways of being. Judaism has gone through a paradigm shift; Christian renewal is just as necessary as Jewish renewal. In this coming aeon we cannot take the tradition without reworking it. We have to renew it, bring it to life, make it a living experience.

If I answer the question, what is God?, I've already made an idol. If I ask, who is God?, then God is the one I stand before who is my reference point in action and consciousness and prayer. God is the one in whom my awareness rests; in other words, I am present in the presence of God, so my mind is not private. Everything that is happening in my head has everything to do with God. My thoughts and feelings are known just as my heart beats, not because I will it but because God makes it beat. My task is simply to collaborate with the Divine purpose.

In each generation the Divine has been seen differently. Most of the language of the synagogue services was modeled on God as a monarch. This model no longer moves or inspires us. One of the renewal issues has to do with feminism. At one point we figured men could run the whole scene. Now we see that without the caring, the nurturing that is in women, the planet will be ravished and may even cease to exist. We cannot interpret God's will if we think God is only male. We have to understand what it means to embrace the feminine aspect of God. The Kabbalah always endorsed this, speaking of the Sh'chinnah as a Divine feminine attribute and presence, but esoteric Judaism as well as many of the other religions ignored it and made God look like an old king with a beard. Now we have to rework it. And whereas before the power was in kings or prophets or in priests or rabbis, now the power has to be with the entire people.

When we become more awake, we begin to discern that our sojourn in the body and on this planet is no accident. We are reminded of the commitment we made to improve the quality of human life on earth and to further the growth of consciousness. When I look at how consciousness moves from a single-celled being or from the big bang, I see that human beings constitute the brain cells of the global brain.

Such thoughts are wake-up thoughts. My daughter said to me, "Papa, when you're asleep, you can wake up, right? But when you're awake, can you wake up even more?" That is such a powerful question. We won't be able to survive unless we wake up even more. The only way to get it together is to get it together. I can't get it together for you; you can't get it together for me. So totalitarianism, in which one dictator or guru gets it together for everyone else, doesn't work any more. We have to learn ways of more meaningful collaboration.

The deepest form of reflection is enlightenment, revelation, self-realization, salvation, to be the one who is born again, to be active in the world's redemption. All the technology for enlightenment is available to us. Yet if we compare our wonderful know-how of that enlightenment virtuosity with our crudeness in the area of harmonious social, political, and economic interaction, we see that our knowledge in the field of peace is little compared to our sophistication in the field of war. People who deal in ethics, philosophy, religion, and morals are still using kindergarten reality maps while scientists are designing destruction with frightening effectiveness with the aid of state-of-the-art computers. Peace and ecology groups compete for publicity and money but know so little about how to collaborate and work together toward improving the quality of life. They haven't gotten it together enough to get it together.

If there were a terrible plague, there is no doubt that biologists the world over would work closely together to find an antidote and vaccination to diminish the ravages of the disease. There would be no difficulty in collaborating. And yet are we not so close to destruction? We are not dealing with biology or immunology but with human motivation, and most of us have little knowledge of how to become effective cooperators for the sake of the survival of our planet.

It is time to realize that mere goodwill and peaceful intentions alone will not do what we must do. We and others who remember we are bodhisattvas, messiahs, mahdis, and avatars have to find a way to create modules of collaboration and effectiveness that will serve as models for others. On reflection, we may become aware that we need most urgently to get together about getting it together.

When we look at the Kabbalah, there are four letters in God's name—YHVH. When we look at these four letters of the Divine, we see a relationship between the religions, between the spiritual paths. Yud is like Raja Yoga, which sees the search for the infinite through the tantric; Heh is like Jyana Yoga, which sees God as the cause not the effect, yet a cause that is always causeless; Vav is like Bhakti Yoga, which sees God as the Divine presence, the mother, and the lover; and the other Heh of the Divine name is like Karma

Yoga, which sees God as present in the law of all things. Our brains are hard-wired on the same gestalt. The reptilian brain is seen in the laws of what we can or can't touch; these reflect the karma aspect. The limbic or devotional aspect is seen in mantra, music, and song. Each religion has a philosophical system—how it sees what it is doing—which is the cortex level. But more than 85 percent of the brain isn't accessible yet, isn't formatted, and that is where our intuition is.

Most synagogues, churches, and so on, are trying to deal with the cortex. This makes them boring. When you come to an African American church and the limbic is alive, then you are in a safe space where you can dance, you can scream, and all those feelings have expression. This means that the limbic has been honored. The reptilian brain is also honored, for then the preacher comes and gives ideas. You get something and the cortex is happy. Peak experiences reside where I meet the holiness in myself, in the transcendent part. We each long to be closer to pure is-ness, to be less in illusion, to be clearer about how we form part of the great whole. I can have more awareness of the great whole beyond my ego, so awakening is invited.

In peace negotiations we always talk to our enemy as if all the enemy had was a forebrain, a cortex. What about the enemy's insecurity? In the Middle East the reptilian brains are fighting. Retaliation begets retaliation, and so the terror grows as we demonize each other. To see the others as human as myself, I need to allow myself to feel with them. Unless somebody cries with the parents and grandparents who have lost children on both sides, unless someone is going to own that he or she has had pain and that they have had pain, the fighting will not stop. Both sides need to know that this experiment of having, ultimately, to share the land, will not be called off; we have to work it out.

People have been treated as invisible but can't be expected to remain invisible. This is one of the reasons why we hear the cry, "We live in the Gaza strip, we are hungry, we live in a hellhole, our children are ill, nothing is working out for us. We live in constant frustration; can't you see that? So what are we going to do if we are not seen or heard? Throw a bomb!" This means all other avenues of expression have failed them. Terrorism isn't going to be neutralized by antiterrorism; it will be reduced by letting the people speak up and be visible. We can't say that Sinn Fein has no right to exist. We can't say that we don't negotiate with Hamas. Saying that these people are invisible, these people are nonhuman, is totally inappropriate; it doesn't work. We must see and hear each other. We must be present for the other people while they unload their anger.

Most Jews have not expressed their anger about the Holocaust. When you come into a Jewish place and you feel a seething underneath, you know that the anger needs to be expressed. We have to create situations in which the expression of anger won't harm other people. Anger is a very powerful thing; it comes out of the belly and it can make us sick. Not until after we have had permission to express anger can we go to the place of lifting it higher. I feel a lot of people ignoring their real feelings, like they are putting spirituality on top of unresolved personal issues or putting whipped cream on top of garbage, and it soon begins to smell.

In the past every religion used to have a belief that the Messiah will come again: Jesus will come again, or the Maitreya Buddha will come again, or the Imam will come again. Then that religion will emerge triumphant and all the other religions will grovel in the dust, saying, "You were right all along and we were wrong." That notion is called triumphalism. However, with the realization of the planet as a living whole, with the emergence of Gaia, every religion is being seen as necessary, just as every organ in the body is necessary. This means that in the same way a species is important, so a religion is important. Judaism may be like the liver, Christianity like the lungs or the brain, and another like the heart. We need them all. When you start saying that only one is triumphant, you are saying there is only the heart, but the heart cannot be sustained without the lungs. The recognition that we need each other is basic to togetherness.

I imagine that when the Jews were on Mount Sinai receiving the Torah there was a great flash of the cosmic presence, of what it's all about, and that we have always sought to recapture that, to celebrate, to get back to that great moment of cosmic insight. So we create the family setting and have intergenerational transmissions. The rule of Shabbas is, "And the children of Israel shall keep the Sabbath," so we make the sabbath for each generation an everlasting covenant, an ever-renewing, ever-regenerating thing. That is what is so important here—the forms that make that experience organically repeatable— like chicken soup on Friday night. There's a warmth in family; you stop bickering so much, you sit around the table, you give each other hugs and blessings, and you repeat this each week.

The hardest, the worst experience that we all have is that the wheel of time is going so fast that none of us gets the chance for reflecting, for rebuilding ourselves, for renewing ourselves. The fabric of family life has been destroyed; television is eating up consciousness. People don't spend time talking or sharing or even eating together. That's why Shabbas is so important. We have to take time out. We have to light the candles on Friday evening and reflect on what the week was all about, turn off the telephone, disconnect ourselves from the media, and share, sing, make music, and tell stories together. We have to renew ourselves and each other.

Most religious systems have been operating on the solitariness of spirituality: I meditate, and when I go into myself, I do it alone. What I like so much about the Jewish contribution is the togetherness of spirituality. I asked somebody what his spiritual way was and he said he had a wonderful path. "I do Yoga, I do Tai Chi, I do meditation." I asked him how often he does it, and he said, "Well, I also need to do quality time with my family, so I don't do it that often." And I asked, "How often do you do quality time with your family?" And he said, "Not often enough; I'm not together enough, I'm not centered enough, I need to do more Yoga to do it." And I said, "Why don't you put it together, do your spiritual path with your family during quality time?" And that is what Shabbas is. It's diving together into quality time. This is socializing the meditative stuff, making it something that is intergenerational, more a way of life. This is called renewal.

We need to give more blessings. The world is underblessed. It is so very important. When you sit down before you have your meal, bless the food and bless your body; say, "Whatever is good for me, let it be absorbed, and whatever is not good for me, let it be released." Bless your life and your loved ones. Let blessings fill your being.

Anne Bancroft

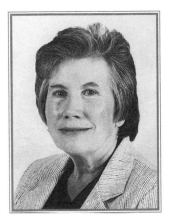

Midway through her life, Anne Bancroft found mysticism to be her direction. Previously an English teacher, she has since written a number of books about the mystical experience as perceived by different people and about the spiritual journey itself. "It is in the living out of the everyday actuality of things in their homeliest detail," she says, "that the mystic can truly experience the many-splendored wonder of this vivid and extraordinary existence."

Everyday Mysticism

Mysticism is a word that can seem so loose and vague, suggesting other worlds and gods and a realm of cosmic mush, that many people avoid using it altogether, tending to despise it. But that's a pity, because the world's languages have very few words to describe any condition that transcends and illuminates ordinary consciousness. *Mysticism* is one that we lose at our peril.

There are many ways of looking at mysticism. Some people vaguely think of it as the life of their own innerness, others as a religious state that is difficult and rather odd—a condition they would find themselves in at the top of some tricky spiritual ladder they have no intention of climbing. And yet others are convinced they know what mysticism is because that's what they feel when they join in a chant or hug a tree.

Each of these interpretations seems to need a bigger framework in which to see things more clearly. The people who believe that mysticism is about themselves, the others who think it is not at all for themselves, and the ones who require special conditions such as a full moon or a sacred site in which to experience it—each needs to move into a larger landscape, one that transcends the narrow boundaries of involvement with the self. That landscape is available here and now, for it is the reality within which we live our lives. If we can look at that reality through the wide-angle lens of objectivity, which gives a farseeing view, rather than through the reading glass lens, which shows up all that is close—our own desires and difficulties, for instance—but blurs everything else, then we will find it easier to understand what mysticism means.

In the wide-angle lens of objectivity, reality, the concrete world in all its marvel, is translucently clear. Seeing it with transcendent clarity is what mysticism means, and it turns out that it's the goal not only of religion but also of everything in our world that points beyond itself—music, poetry, art, selfless action. Whether we see things in a mystical way or not makes no difference to the reality, but it makes a very great difference to us. We are not fully human, not complete or real, until our lives come to be based on the consciousness of a vastly deep meaning that lies enfolded in the world of the everyday and until we turn our attention to that reality as the most necessary and vital nourishment.

And this is more than easy because there are plenty of things in ordinary normal experience that point to its existence, to its "it-ness." There are the sudden impacts of beauty that we all feel—the flowering branch of cherry, the elegant symmetry of a cat, the moving clouds—and a thousand other small or big sights that come into being, filled with timelessness and infinity as soon as we put our undivided attention on them. We use our sense of sight to see them, but we are witnessing a wonder that goes beyond sense.

Then there are the moments when it seems as though our lives are not bounded only by heredity and environment and all the interconnecting causes of our physical existence but are touching some other, deeper power. There is the unexpected opportunity, the path that suddenly opens up in front of us, the things we feel compelled to say or do in spite of ourselves, the essential contact with a person we have never heard of before. It seems as though quite often there is a personal directing power, a hand on the shoulder, that is working through circumstances to push us in certain directions, and the more we are aware of it, the easier it is to follow it in our lives.

None of this stands up to any materialistic analysis. No strict scientist would bother with it for a minute. In fact, this is where mysticism begins to get its bad name, for it implies that there are unsuspected realms of consciousness within the universe which the materialist knows nothing of, and materialism will have none of that. The materialist sees the surface of life and is content with it. But many people find themselves aware of a depth and mystery to their existence, a richer and more truthful reality behind the world of everyday sense that seems a profoundly spiritual force, beckoning them to experience it, to taste it with their own being.

It's quite easy to avoid this whole challenge, because it seems hidden and inward and most people are far too busy keeping up with their lives in an outward way to want to bother with it. But if we do begin to take it seriously, we begin to see that no understanding of life on this earth is complete without it. Surely it means that we and all the rest of existence are essentially spiritual, as much as we are animal, and that if we want to find a way of ultimate fulfillment, in which we are able to bring to fruition all the possibilities in ourselves, we must be in touch not only with our bodies and minds but also with that sense of timeless and infinite mystery that is the deepest part of our consciousness.

The significance of being human is that we have choice. We can choose to ignore anything that calls us to greater effort. Or we can begin to accept that the meaning of our life is bound up with the whole mystery of the universe. Then life itself is enhanced, for all reality comes to be seen in a new light. Each of the everyday practical things we do is enriched by a sense of ultimate meaning that brings calmness and coherence. Usually we are in a state of endless unrest, believing our lives to consist of either gaining and having or discarding and rejecting. Constantly craving and clutching, we lose sight of the state of being altogether. But when the mystical understanding of depth and otherness is there, the horizon widens and all our cravings and rejections are seen in proportion, seen with steadiness and put in their own scale of time and place rather than occupying the whole of our attention.

Many people in our day seem helpless, unable to make sense of their lives, and full of fears about the future. They have no hold on the infinite, no freedom from time and place. They are lacking a feeling of inner security which comes from a sense of meaning and purpose. This is not to say that they live in an actual and practical world and that the mystic somehow escapes this world. Rather, it is in the living out of the everyday actuality of things in their homeliest detail and with all their demands that the mystic can truly experience the many-splendored wonder of this vivid and extraordinary existence, that he or she can fully feel the mystery of consciousness that pervades the universe. But without that hold on the infinite, all the everyday situations we encounter often bring confusion, worry, unsteadiness, and despair. When they are seen in the light of an objective clarity—abstract words perhaps but which do, when experienced, bring a sense of personal and loving security—our confusion falls away. Suffering remains, but not in the same muddled helpless way.

There was a time when religions wanted to instill this loving security. But perhaps it more truly belongs to evolution itself. As we grow out of our need to clutch at and depend on a religion, so we will feel the freedom of our deep drive toward an ever and ever clearer reality. This is a movement of the spirit to which we may well be already adapted, as a bird is to the air.

The reality itself is prodding us, encouraging us to take off and try our wings. And because we are born this way, with this inborn human ability to grow and be transformed in the process, we can see that there is no cause for self-importance but only for a humble joy in the process.

So religion may no longer be the path to take, although in the origins of each religion is a commitment to the transcendent and a confident dependence on its existence. This confidence and commitment bring the abundant life often talked about in all the scriptures, and leading there is the "invisible path, beyond the tracing of gods or men"—the path which goes beyond all religions and which brings us to the "perfect joy" of Nirvana.

This means that when we think of our own lives, we can see that the spiritual aspect of them is not a fenced-off area with its own special thoughts and feelings of devotion which needs to be carefully shielded from the rough and tumble of the oh-so-ordinary world. Nor is it a replacement, a specialized and difficult alternative, for our usual practical life. It is quite the opposite. The taking of the path, the spiritual journey, the discovery of the meaning of our lives, give everything we do in ordinary life a significance and quality that it would not otherwise have.

Nor does treading the path mean that I am constantly gazing at my own thoughts, attending to the condition of my soul, and noting all my own reactions, dreams, and so on, as though studying the workings is going to lead me to the answer. Many of us do this, having inherited such an attitude from the physicist Newton, who believed that the nature of the whole could be found by analyzing the parts. But in our day there is a new physics which has shown us that the whole is always more and other than the sum of its parts and that finding the whole will lead us more surely to understanding the parts properly.

So although some hard work may be needed at the beginning when our thoughts are dictated by misunderstandings and ignorance and when they splinter and scatter in every direction in such a way that we have to deal with ourselves before we can do anything else, yet we should not remain in-turned. The path itself always leads away from the narrowness of an ego-bound life to a free and creative and loving existence in which the link is felt with every other creature in the world.

To become fully alive and fully human and to take our proper evolutionary place in the cosmos means a continual give and take with the reality in which we live and move and have our being. Just as our lungs need air and our bodies need nourishment, all of which we gather from our surrounding environment, so our spirits need contact with that which is their true natures in the same organic way that our bodies need food. We need to feed on the infinite reality that is never absent, even if we are not always aware of it.

There are many ways in which we can do this. We live in an age when dogma cannot any more suppress the longings of the mystic and many people have found their path to be in meditation or ritual, Eastern or Western. If the motivation is right, it scarcely matters what we do. If all our actions are dedicated to living in this amazing moment, with all its sights and sounds for the joy of our senses and all its challenges and responsibilities for the growth of our personality, then we are fully on the path wherever we are.

This means that all those anxious moments of wondering what is the best thing to do for oneself or even what is the most helpful way of life for humanity can be encompassed in one question: what function should my life fulfill within the great and mysterious evolution of existence? Immediately we are then part of the whole and not an isolated self. And if we are open to the magnetism of that mystery, we will feel the subtle pressures of direction which move us in ways that we may not have envisioned before.

A lot of our confusion arises from trying to place the spiritual and the practical aspects of our lives into separate compartments instead of seeing them as belonging to one whole. If our practical lives are full of ourselves—what we own, what we want to do or to have, worries about our health and about our importance or our rights, and ambitions for success—we are not suddenly going to find a spiritual life that is different from that list. Everything will go on in the same old way as long as the self is the center. It is only when the center is shifted altogether, when objective clarity lights the scene and we see once and for all that the center is not only within us but is a great and wide consciousness that embraces everything, that a sense of awakening takes place and we move thankfully into a new center of realization.

"All things were in Nirvana from the very beginning," said the Buddha. Within this world, within this space of ourselves, within this very moment, we can discover Nirvana and recognize it and live from it, and so do all we are asked to do as a total fulfillment of how we are meant to be.

Contributor Biographies

DR. A. T. ARIYARATNE   Having formulated an innovative model for individual and communal upliftment, Dr. Ariyaratne founded the Sarvodaya Shramadana Movement in Sri Lanka, the world's largest nongovernment movement for people's progress, affecting over 10, 000 villages. He has written six volumes of collected works, won international acclaim as a social scientist, and received numerous awards including the Mahatma Gandhi Peace Prize in 1996. He was a president of the World Parliament of Religions in 1993, and an international president of the World Conference on Religion and Peace in 1994.

ANNE BANCROFT   A profound mystical experience transformed Anne's life in her forties and led her to write a number of books about it: *The Spiritual Journey, Weavers of Wisdom, Women in Search of the Sacred, Twentieth Century Mystics and Sages,* as well as books about Buddhism and medieval mystics. She teaches at the Sharpham College for Buddhist Studies.

STEPHEN AND MARTINE BATCHELOR   Stephen was a monk in Buddhist monasteries in India, Switzerland, and Korea and is now director of studies of the Sharpham College for Buddhist Studies in Devon, England. He is the author of many books, including *The Awakening of the West* and *Buddhism Without Beliefs.* Martine was a Zen Buddhist nun in Korea for ten years and now leads meditation retreats. She is the author of *Walking on Lotus Flowers* and co-editor of *Buddhism and Ecology.*

JOHN BIRD   The *Big Issue* street newspaper in London was launched by John in 1991; it offers a chance for homeless people to earn a living and reestablish their lives. He is now editor-in-chief of *Big Issue* and a trustee of the Big Issue Foundation which offers guidance, support, and training in numerous skills. In recognition of his work for the homeless, John was awarded a Member of the British Empire by Queen Elizabeth in 1995.

SHEILA CASSIDY, M.D.   A doctor since 1963, Sheila was detained and tortured in Chile in 1971 for treating a wounded revolutionary. Returning to England, she was appointed medical director of Saint Luke's Hospice in Plymouth and later became palliative care specialist at Plymouth General Hospital. She is presently psychosocial oncologist in the Plymouth Cancer Center, where she provides psychosocial care for cancer patients. She is the author of many books, including *Audacity to Believe, Sharing the Darkness,* and *The Loneliest Journey.*

H.H. THE DALAI LAMA   The fourteenth Dalai Lama of Tibet is both spiritual and temporal leader of the Tibetan people. In 1959 he escaped from Tibet to India, following the Chinese invasion and ruthless suppression of the Tibetan people and their culture. He has successfully led the Tibetan refugees to rehabilitation and the preservation of their unique culture. His constant advocacy of nonviolence led to his being awarded the Nobel Peace Prize in 1989. He is recognized by governments and heads of state worldwide. He is the author of many books, including *My Land, My People* and *Freedom in Exile.*

RAM DASS   In the early sixties, with Timothy Leary and others, Ram Dass (Richard Alpert) researched the use of psychedelics as an agent for exploring human consciousness. He then went to India and met his teacher, Neem Karoli Baba, who emphasized service to others. He founded the Hanuman Foundation in 1974 and has since taught internationally about the nature of consciousness and service as a spiritual path. He is considered by many to be one of the foremost spiritual teachers in the West. He is the author of numerous books, including *Be Here Now, Grist for the Mill, How Can I Help?,* and *Compassion in Action.*

CHRISTINA FELDMAN   Cofounder and guiding teacher at Gaia House Retreat Centre in England and a guiding teacher at the Insight Meditation Society in Barre, Massachusetts, Christina has been leading insight meditation retreats since 1976. She is the author of *Women Awake* and *Quest of the Warrior Woman* and coauthor with Jack Kornfield of *Soul Food.*

RICK FIELDS   Former editor of *New Age Journal* and current editor-in-chief of *Yoga Journal,* Rick is the author of *How the Swans Came to the Lake; Chop Wood, Carry Water;* and *The Code of the Warrior.*

MATTHEW FOX   An ordained priest since 1967 and founder of the Institute in Culture and Creation Spirituality, Matthew is the president of the University of Creation Spirituality in Oakland, California. He is the author of many books, including *Original Blessing, The Reinvention of Work,* and his autobiography, *Confessions: The Making of a Postdenominational Priest.* He was awarded the Courage of Conscience Award by the Peace Abbey of Sherborn, Massachusetts.

MILLARD FULLER   Millard is the founder, along with his wife, Linda, and president of Habitat for Humanity International, a worldwide Christian housing ministry in Georgia. More that 250, 000 people now have safe and affordable housing due to Habitat's work. Millard has written six books about Habitat for Humanity, including *A Simple, Decent Place to Live* and *The Theology of the Hammer.* He received the Presidential Medal of Freedom in 1996, was voted Builder of the Year in 1995 by *Professional Builder* magazine, and received the Martin Luther King, Jr., Award. He and Linda were awarded the 1994 Harry S. Truman Public Service Award.

PETER GOLDFARB   An award-winning producer, director, and actor in theater, television, and film, Peter is a founding faculty member of the Naropa Institute and guest artist at the University of Colorado. He teaches at the Circle in the Square in New York City and is a director of the Eugene O'Neill Theater Center and of the International Theater Institute in the United States. He recently received the Best Actor of 1996 Award from *Dramalogue Magazine*.

MIKHAIL GORBACHEV   Elected as general secretary of the Soviet Union in 1985 and chairman in 1989, he became the first democratically elected president of the Soviet Union in 1990. Mikhail is credited with *peristroika*—the restructuring of the economy—and with *glasnost*—openness in political and cultural affairs. He brought about the social transformation of the U.S.S.R., for which he won the Nobel Peace Prize in 1990. He is the founder of the Foundation for Social, Economic, and Political Research in Moscow, known as the Gorbachev Foundation.

THICH NHAT HANH   Born in Vietnam and a Zen Buddhist monk since the age of sixteen, he is the founder of Plum Village, a retreat community in southwestern France. He was nominated for the Nobel Peace Prize by Martin Luther King, Jr., for his work to stop the Vietnam war. He is an international teacher and the best-selling author of more than seventy books, including *Being Peace, Peace Is Every Step, Love in Action,* and *Old Path White Clouds: Walking in the Footsteps of the Buddha.*

PAUL HAWKEN   Businessperson and environmentalist and founder of Smith & Hawken, the U.S. garden retail and catalogue company, Paul is chairman of The Natural Step, a nonprofit educational foundation dedicated to guiding society toward a sustainable future. He is the author of many books, including *The Next Economy, Growing a Business* (made into a seventeen part PBS television series), and *The Ecology of Commerce.* He has received the Small Business Administration Entrepreneur of the Year Award, the Utne 100 Award in 1995, and the Council on Economic Priorities Environmental Stewardship Award.

WILL KEEPIN   Will is an environmental scientist and co-director of the Shavano Institute in Boulder, Colorado, a nonprofit organization that sponsors Leading with Spirit, a training program in transformational leadership for social change professionals. Formerly consulting physicist to the Energy Foundation, he is on the adjunct faculty of the California Institute of Integral Studies and is consulting editor of *ReVision.*

GENERAL JACK KIDD   A major general in the U.S. Air Force, now retired, Jack was deeply involved in starting, fighting, operating, and ending three of America's five major wars this century. He was also involved in planning several more, including World War III. He is now applying his experience to strengthen the United Nations to end all wars of aggression. He is the recipient of many awards and decorations, including the Distinguished Service Medal, the Silver Star, the Distinguished Flying Cross, and the Air Force Commendation Medal.

GLENYS KINNOCK   Elected to the European Parliament in 1994 and representative of the South Wales East constituency, Glenys is president of One World Action, the development NGO. She is also vice president of the Africa

Caribbean and Pacific/European Union Joint Assembly, a member of the Human Rights Subcommittee, and vice president of Steel Action in the European Parliament in Brussels.

KITARO   A contemporary Japanese musician who pioneered an evolutionary music that crosses classical, jazz, and pop, Kitaro has made more than sixteen albums and sold more than ten million copies worldwide.

KITTISARO AND THANISSARA   Kittisaro (Randolph Weinberg) was on a Rhodes scholarship to Oxford when he went to Thailand. There he became a Buddhist monk with Ajahn Chah, the renown Thai teacher. He later helped to establish the Theravada forest monasteries in England. He disrobed after fifteen years. Thanissara (Mary Peacock) trained as a Buddhist nun for twelve years under the guidance of Ajahn Chah and Ajahn Sumedho. Now married, Kittisaro and Thanissara are resident teachers at the Ixopo Buddhist Retreat Center in South Africa.

SATISH KUMAR   After nine years as a Jain monk, at the age of eighteen Satish walked the length of India, persuading landlords to donate land to the landless. He gathered approximately five million acres as gifts to the poor. He then walked from India to the United States for peace. He has edited and published *Resurgence* magazine since 1974, founded the Small School in Hartland, Devon, in 1982, and the Schumacher College in Dartington, England, an international center of study informed by ecological and spiritual values. He is the founder of Green Books and the author of *No Destination*.

WINONA LADUKE   A longtime environmentalist and indigenous rights activist, Winona was vice presidential running mate to Ralph Nader for the Green Party in the U.S. 1996 elections. She is program director of the Seventh Generation Fund's Environmental Program and campaign director of the White Earth Land Recovery Project. She won the Reebok Human Rights Award in 1988, was named in 1994 one of *Time* magazine's Fifty for the Future: Leaders in America Under 40 Years of Age, and was selected for the Thomas Merton Award in 1996.

STEPHEN LEVINE   Meditation teacher and past director of the Hanuman Foundation Dying Project, Stephen, with his wife, Ondrea, has been deeply involved in enabling the terminally ill and their loved ones to find their healing. He is the best-selling author of many books, including *Healing into Life and Death, Who Dies?, Embracing the Beloved,* and *A Year to Live.*

BO LOZOFF   The founder, with his wife, Sita, of the Prison-Ashram Project, Bo has helped prisoners and prison staff throughout the world to use their harsh environment to develop kindness and compassion. Their newsletter, "A Little Good News," reaches more than 30,000 prisoners and ex-prisoners, and his book, *We're All Doing Time,* is given free to any prisoner who requests it. Director of the Human Kindness Foundation in North Carolina, he has led hundreds of workshops in prisons and universities.

HELENA NORBERG-HODGE   Helena is founder and director of the International Society for Ecology and Culture, the Ladakh Project, and the Ladakh Ecological Development Group (LEDeG). Helena and LEDeG received the Right Livelihood Award in 1986. She is the author of *Ancient Futures: Learning from Ladakh,* and has lectured extensively to parliamentarians in Germany, Sweden, and England, at the White House, and to the U.S. Congress, UNESCO, and the World Bank.

YOKO ONO   Artist, poet, musician, with paintings and sculptures in galleries worldwide, Yoko won the Grammy Award in 1981 for Album of the Year, with husband John Lennon, for *Double Fantasy.*

DEAN ORNISH, M.D.   Dean is president of the Preventive Medicine Research Institute in California, clinical professor of medicine at the University of California, director of the Integrative Medicine Center, and attending physician at the California Pacific Medical Center in the United States. Dean was selected as one of the most interesting people of 1995 by *People* magazine and as one of the fifty most outstanding members of his generation by *Life* magazine. He is the author of four best-selling books, including *Dr. Dean Ornish's Program for Reversing Heart Disease* and *Stress, Diet, and Your Heart.*

JILL PURCE   Interested in the spiritual properties of the voice, Jill worked with the composer Karlheinz Stockhausen, learned Mongolian and Tibetan overtone chanting, and studied with the chantmaster of the Gyutö Tibetan Monastery and Tantric College. She teaches diverse forms of sacred chant internationally and is the author of *The Mystic Spiral.*

RACHEL NAOMI REMEN, M.D.   Medical director of the Commonweal Cancer Help Program and director and founder of the Institute for the Study of Health and Illness at Commonweal, which is accredited by the California Medical Association, Rachel is associate clinical professor of family and community medicine at the UCSF School of Medicine and director of the UCSF Medical School course "The Healer's Art." She is the author of the bestseller *Kitchen Table Wisdom: Stories That Heal,* winner of the 1996 Wilbur Award.

ANITA RODDICK   Anita founded The Body Shop, which now has approximately 1,400 branches in 45 countries, and is committed to animal protection, environmental protection, and respect for human rights. She is an international leader in the business world, where she advocates safe environmental standards, and is known for her numerous campaigns for human rights around the world. She has won many awards, including Philanthropist of the Year in 1996 from the Institute of Charitable Fundraising Managers in the United Kingdom, and received an Order of the British Empire in 1988.

SRI SWAMI SATCHIDANANDA   Swamiji was a student of Ramana Maharshi and Sri Swami Sivananda and founded Integral Yoga institutes worldwide and the Satchidananda Ashram and Lotus Temple in Virginia. The author of many books, including *The Living Gita* and *The Golden Present,* Swamiji travels extensively as a messenger of peace. He is the recipient of many humanitarian awards, including the Martin Buber Award for Outstanding Service to Humanity.

RABBI ZALMAN SCHACHTER-SHALOMI   Ordained as a rabbi in 1947 by the Lubavitch Yeshivah in Brooklyn, Reb Zalman has been at the forefront of pioneering Jewish spiritual renewal. He is professor emeritus of Temple University; holder of the World Wisdom Chair at Naropa Institute, Boulder, Colorado; and founder of the Spiritual Eldering Institute. He has been a spiritual guide for countless Jews and non-Jews. He is the author of *Spiritual Intimacy, Paradigm Shift,* and *From Age-ing to Sage-ing.*

RUPERT SHELDRAKE   Biochemist, teacher, and Fellow of Clare College, Cambridge, England, Rupert has spent his life in fascination of nature and the connection between science and spirituality. He is known for his development of the idea of morphic resonance, the author of *The Rebirth of Nature, A New Science of Life,* and *Seven Experiments That Could Change the World,* and the coauthor of two books of dialogue with Matthew Fox: *Natural Grace* and *The Physics of Angels.*

BERNIE SIEGEL, M.D.   Now a retired pediatric and general surgeon, Bernie started Exceptional Cancer Patients (ECap) in 1978, based on "carefrontation"—a loving, safe, and therapeutic confrontation that facilitates personal change and healing. He is involved in humanizing medical education and making the medical profession aware of the mind-body connection. He is the best-selling author of *Love, Medicine, and Miracles; Peace, Love, and Healing;* and *How to Live Between Office Visits: A Guide to Life, Love, and Health.*

SULAK SIVARAKSA   A social activist and founder of many initiatives that seek to combat consumer values and promote spiritually based development, Sulak has had his work repeatedly repressed by the Thai authorities. He created the *Social Science Review,* which soon became the most influential publication in Thailand; a string of social welfare and development organizations; the famous Jungle University for fleeing Burmese students; and a new college in Thailand: the Spirit in Education Movement.

CATHRINE SNEED   A county sheriff for many years, Cathrine is the founder of the San Francisco County Jail Horticulture Program and the director of the Garden Project. Cathrine combined her experience as a jail counselor and her horticulture and legal training to teach prisoners to grow food and then supply seniors, homeless people, and AIDS victims. Recipient of many awards, including the Hero of the Earth Award by the Eddie Bauer Corporation, she has lectured internationally on the Garden Project.

HANNE STRONG   Hanne is president of Manitou Foundation, founded in 1988, and Manitou Institute. These organizations are establishing an ecumenical and sustainable teaching community in the United States. She is founder of the Earth Restoration Corps, an international educational program for youth and adults to restore and sustain the earth, and has worked extensively with nonprofit organizations for Native Americans, the handicapped, and street children in both Kenya and New York.

ROBERT THURMAN   Previously a Buddhist monk, Robert is now Jey Tsong Khapa Professor of Indo-Tibetan Studies at Columbia University, New York, and was listed as one of *Time* magazine's fifty most influential people in 1997. He is an outspoken supporter of the Dalai Lama and the Tibetan struggle for freedom and is president of Tibet House New York. Robert is the author of many books, including *Inner Revolution: Life, Liberty, and the Pursuit of Real Happiness* and *The Tibetan Book of the Dead*.

CHRISTOPHER TITMUSS   Cofounder and guiding teacher of Gaia House Retreat Center, Devon, England, he teaches insight meditation retreats worldwide. A former Buddhist monk in Thailand and India, he is a founding member of the international board of the Buddhist Peace Fellowship. His books include *The Green Buddha* and *The Profound and the Profane,* and *Light on Enlightenment.*

ARCHBISHOP DESMOND TUTU   A priest since 1961, Desmond Tutu became bishop of Lesotho in 1975. After the Soweto uprising in 1976, he became general secretary of the South African Council of Churches, known as a prominent antiapartheid figure, and recognized as the leader of the crusade for justice and reconciliation. He received the Nobel Peace Prize in 1984 for this work. In 1986 he was elected archbishop of Cape Town; now retired as archbishop, he has been named archbishop emeritus of South Africa. He chairs the Truth and Reconciliation Commission in South Africa and is considered one of the few people who have the standing to effect racial reconciliation.

RAMA VERNON   Nearly 10,000 Soviet and American citizens have participated in programs sponsored by the Center for International Dialogue, founded by Rama in 1984. She has initiated Soviet-American Citizens Summits; dialogues between former Soviet Republics and in the Middle East, Ethiopia, Central America, and Africa; and a series of Arab-American dialogues during the Gulf War. She is the founder of Women of Vision and Action and of *Yoga Journal* magazine. She was the recipient of the 1991 Inside Edge Foundation World Peace Award and the Evart T. Loomis World Peace Award.

RUBY WAX   Entertainer, writer, and actress, Ruby spent many years with the Royal Shakespeare Company, during which time she wrote *Desperately Yours,* which became an off-Broadway hit. She is best known for her unusual television documentaries and interviews, including *Ruby Takes a Trip, East Meets Wax, The Full Wax,* and *Ruby's Health Quest.* She has worked with Dawn French and Jennifer Saunders on two series of *Girls on Top.*

MARIANNE WILLIAMSON   A Unity Church minister and an international lecturer in spirituality and new thought, Marianne is the best-selling author of *A Return to Love, A Woman's Worth, The Healing of America,* and a children's book, *Emma and Mommy Talk to God*. She has done extensive charitable work throughout the United States in service to people with life-challenging illnesses.

MUHAMMAD YUNUS Professor of economics at Chittagong University, Bangladesh, and director of the Rural Economics Program until 1989, Muhammad founded the Grameen Bank in 1976. He is currently the managing director of the bank. A member of numerous international advisory committees, he is the recipient of many awards, including the US Humanitarian Award 1993, the US Pfeffer Peace Prize 1994, the Swiss Max Schmidheiny Foundation Freedom Prize 1995, and the US International Activist Award 1997, all in recognition of his work in creating a banking system that has given millions of the most impoverished access to adequate food and housing for the first time in their lives.

About the Editors

EDDIE AND DEBBIE SHAPIRO are respected spiritual teachers and international workshop leaders. They are the authors of many books, including *Peace Within the Stillness, Clear Mind Open Heart, Out of Your Mind—The Only Place to Be!* and editors of *The Way Ahead.* Eddie, from New York City, trained as a swami in India with Paramahamsa Satyananda. He is the author of *Inner Conscious Relaxation.* Debbie, from England, trained in Buddhist meditation, bodywork, and bodymind therapy. She is the author of *Your Body Speaks Your Mind* and *The Bodymind Workbook.* They live in England and the United States.